Take Control of Your Health

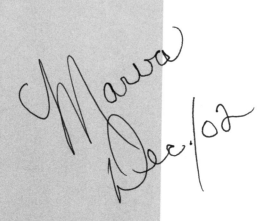

Take Control of Your Health

A WOMAN'S GUIDE TO STAYING WELL AT ANY AGE

EDITED BY JULIA HANSEN

Rodale Press, Inc.
Emmaus, Pennsylvania

This book is being published simultaneously as *Headlines in Women's Health 1996*.

Copyright © 1996 by Rodale Press, Inc.

Illustrations copyright © 1995 by Liz Grace

The credits for this book begin on page 289.

Library of Congress Cataloging-in-Publication Data

Take control of your health: a woman's guide to staying well at any
  age / edited by Julia Hansen.
        p.   cm.
    Includes index.
    ISBN 0–87596–336–6   paperback
    1. Women—Health and hygiene.   2. Women—Mental health.
  3. Women—Nutrition.   I. Hansen, Julia.
  RA778.T345, 1995
  613'.04244—dc20

Distributed in the book trade by St. Martin's Press

2   4   6   8   10   9   7   5   3   1   paperback

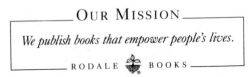

_____ OUR MISSION _____

We publish books that empower people's lives.

_____ RODALE ❦ BOOKS _____

Take Control of Your Health Editorial Staff

Contributing Writers: **Maureen Boland, Pamela Boyer, Jan Bresnick, Lisa Delaney, Denise Foley, Greg Gutfeld, Rosemary Iconis, Jeff Meade, Ellen Michaud, Marty Munson, Eileen Nechas, Gail North, Lynn O'Shaughnessy, Cathy Perlmutter, Maureen Sangiorgio, Maggie Spilner, Michele Stanten, Elisabeth Torg, Linda Villarosa, Therese Walsh**
Editor: **Julia Hansen**
Managing Editor: **Sharon Faelten**
Permissions Coordinator: **Anita Small**
Associate Art Director, Cover Designer: **Faith Hague**
Book Designer: **Joyce C. Weston**
Illustrator: **Liz Grace**
Studio Manager: **Joe Golden**
Technical Artists: **Kristen Morgan Downey, David Q. Pryor**
Page Composition: **Miriam Adkins**
Copy Editor: **Amy K. Fisher**
Production Manager: **Helen Clogston**
Manufacturing Coordinator: **Melinda B. Rizzo**
Office Staff: **Roberta Mulliner, Julie Kehs, Bernadette Sauerwine, Mary Lou Stephen**

Rodale Health and Fitness Books

Vice-President and Editorial Director: **Debora T. Yost**
Art Director: **Jane Colby Knutila**
Research Manager: **Ann Gossy Yermish**
Copy Manager: **Lisa D. Andruscavage**

Contents

PART FIVE: *B*ODY-SHAPING

PART SIX: *A*GE-DEFYING BEAUTY SECRETS

PART SEVEN: *L*OVE AND INTIMACY

PART EIGHT: *S*TRESS CONTROL

Introduction

Your Health Is in Your Hands

Heart disease kills more women than breast cancer, but often goes undetected until it becomes severe.

About 25 percent of all hysterectomies are unnecessary.

Forty percent of women haven't had a Pap smear—the first line of defense against cervical cancer—in the past three years.

Yet such grim statistics belie the encouraging truth: There's a revolution occurring in women's health, and the front lines are dominated by women themselves.

Women are learning about their bodies, questioning the quality of their health care and insisting that health care providers address their unique concerns—concerns that, until recently, tended to be overlooked.

And the medical establishment, along with the government, is listening.

The women's health movement has been gathering force for decades. But its crusade for more and better health care went largely unheeded until the mid-1980s and early 1990s.

The Women's Health Initiative (WHI) is one impetus for the exploding interest in women's health. Launched in 1992, the WHI—a 15-year study involving 160,000 women—is currently the largest clinical trial ever undertaken in the United States. The study is being conducted by the National Institutes of Health in Bethesda, Maryland, and is focusing on how best to prevent and treat heart disease and cancer in women. While both of these conditions strike women as hard as they do men, they had long been regarded as "men's diseases," even by women.

The WHI is also researching the causes of and treatments for osteoporosis. This bone-thinning disease strikes a disproportionate number of older women, restricting their activity and quality of life.

Yet another crucial milestone in women's health occurred in 1993, when the Food and Drug Administration (FDA) recommended that women be represented in drug trials. Until then, the FDA had recommended excluding pregnant women and women of childbearing potential from most of these trials. According to a recent survey by the Pharmaceutical Manufacturers Association, 301 medicines are in development for diseases that affect only women or disproportionately affect women, including heart disease, cancer, stroke, arthritis and osteoporosis.

But the current tidal wave of medical research and government commitment to women's health is only part of the story. Equally important is that women themselves are taking advantage of each new discovery to strengthen their bodies and enhance their quality of life.

Take weight loss, for example. According to recent research, there's no compelling evidence that yo-yo dieting—the repeated weight loss and gain many dieters experience—is worse than being overweight, as has commonly been reported. Another less critical (but no less fascinating) finding: Women's seemingly inborn craving for chocolate and other sweets may have a physiological or hormonal basis. So indulging in a piece of chocolate now and then may actually help women avoid the binges that lead to weight gain.

Or thyroid disease. Experts estimate that eight million Americans have some sort of thyroid disease—which can cause a variety of vague yet troublesome symptoms, including fatigue, weight gain and sleep disturbances—and that the condition is seven times more prevalent in women than in men. Yet it's a simple matter to detect and treat thyroid disease—if a woman knows what to look for.

Or getting older. As many forty- and fiftysomething women already know (and younger women will eventually learn), menopause isn't the stigma it used to be. So it's practical and empowering to learn what to expect from menopause and how to ease the physical and emotional symptoms that may arise.

But as important as these medical issues are, a woman is more than a sum of her parts. As many experts in women's health have long contended, looking good and feeling loved, valued and productive can have a significant effect on a woman's physical and emotional well-being. So can learning to take time for herself.

The purpose of this book—the only annual review of emerging concerns in women's health—is to put the latest news and breakthroughs in women's health into women's hands—*your* hands. Within its pages, you'll find sorely needed information on a multitude of topics that affect both your body and your soul. You'll discover the latest expert-recommended strategies that can help you stay well at any age; eat for good health; slim down and tone up; tap into age-defying health and beauty secrets; and more. This year's issue even contains a special section on stress management to help you meet the many demands on your time and energy.

This book can help give you an instant grasp of some of the most compelling stories in women's health. You'll most likely find yourself turning to this health "almanac" throughout the year. But most importantly, this book is a blueprint for better health that can *help you help yourself*. It can help you target and eliminate lifestyle behaviors that put you at risk, inspire you to de-fat your diet, start an exercise program or reduce the stress in your life.

There's more information about women's health, and more opportunity to access it, than ever before. We at *Prevention* Health Books believe the information in this book can enhance your life. Use it in good health.

Julia Hansen

—JULIA HANSEN, EDITOR

PART ONE

Health Flash

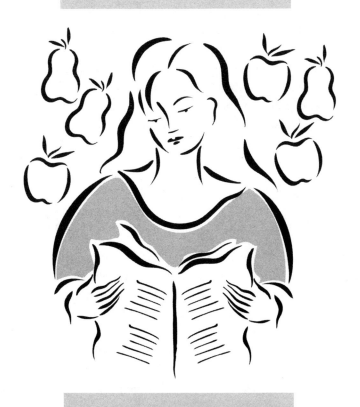

Vegetarian Eating Boom by End of Century

*T*ake out your crystal ball and predict what food trends lie ahead as we enter the twenty-first century. That's what 265 registered dietitians were asked to do in a recent survey. Among their more interesting predictions:

- Expect to see more fusion between ethnic foods—combinations like moo shu pork burritos, pitas stuffed with pizza fixings, and potato skins served with salsa—as ethnic populations flourish in the United States.
- Vegetarianism will become even trendier, especially among Generation X-ers.
- Consumers will be interested less in what's being taken *out* of food (calories, fat, sugar) and more in what's being put *in* (vitamins, minerals and antioxidants).
- Pork and beef growers will continue to breed leaner animals and to position their meat as a "healthy" alternative to chicken.
- Ordering groceries and meals over TV sets will go mainstream, thanks to emerging communications technology.

Dreams May Foretell Ill Health

*C*an dreams warn you that you're about to become ill? According to a handful of researchers, the answer may be yes.

The "scientific" explanation is that each cell in the body can detect minor chemical abnormalities. The subconscious supposedly picks up the body's self-diagnosis and incorporates it in dreams. Although there is no direct evidence of this phenomenon, studies indicate that many people who are ailing have an increased ability to recall dreams, and those dreams are sometimes filled with violent and traumatic imagery, according to Robert L. Van de Castle, Ph.D., author of *Our Dreaming Mind*. If full-blown illness affects your dreams, perhaps changes that occur in the body prior to any outward signs of illness can too. There is anecdotal evidence of the same kind of traumatic dreams occurring well before a malady occurs, sometimes up to a year in advance.

So how do you know whether your nightmares are just that or harbingers of ill health? Clearly, it's easier to tell by reconstructing dream messages after you've been ill. But it is possible to get some clues in advance if you pay attention, says Boston-area hypnotherapist Linda Chalmer Zemel. "If someone in your dream is putting out a house fire with an extinguisher or fixing a flat tire on your car, it may be a sign that the immune system is working hard to fight off an infection. The house and car are frequently symbols of the body," she says. Keeping a journal of your dreams will help you get in the habit of listening to your sleeping self. And if you keep dreaming of a house afire or a flat tire, you may want to schedule a checkup with your doctor.

Ibuprofen Preempts Menstrual Migraines

For the thousands of women whose menstrual cycles are literally a headache, relief may come in a surprisingly humble bottle. It's possible that strategic use of anti-inflammatories may scrub menstruation-related migraines before they even get started.

One of the country's foremost headache experts and executive director of the National Headache Foundation in Chicago, Seymour Diamond, M.D., has tested this strategy on 400 women with menstrual migraines: They take a nonsteroidal anti-inflammatory drug (NSAID), such as naproxen, nabumetone or ibuprofen, two or three days before the onset of their periods and continue it until their periods stop.

Women on the Pill (a known headache exacerbator) used an

expanded form of this preventive strategy: They started the NSAIDs on the 19th day of the Pill cycle and continued them until the day after their periods stopped. An unpublished study of these two strategies found that there were fewer menstrual-related migraines in about 80 percent of the women who tried them.

"The change in hormone levels that occurs with menstruation is probably the most common migraine trigger there is," says Dr. Diamond. Taking NSAIDs could be a simple way to tame that trigger, although researchers can't yet say they know the ins and outs of how (or if) these might block the head-busting hurts. This therapy may also eliminate the need for some of the more heavy-duty medications that are used once a migraine has started.

Head-healing dosages will probably be stronger than what the product label advises, so Dr. Diamond says you can't self-medicate— you have to check with your doctor before you try this technique.

Staying on Schedule Thwarts Weekend Headaches

Do headaches spoil your days off? They could be caused by the abrupt shift from your weekday patterns of eating, sleeping and other activities. Head off weekend headaches by recognizing— and correcting—these common day-off triggers.

Caffeine withdrawal. If your four-cups-a-day habit at work becomes a leisurely single cup at Saturday morning brunch, you may get a caffeine-withdrawal headache. Keep caffeine intake constant throughout the week, recommends Ronald Kaiser, Ph.D., co-director of the Comprehensive Headache Center in Philadelphia. Instead of increasing your weekend intake to equal that during the week, Dr. Kaiser recommends cutting back (gradually, over the course of several weeks) to one or two cups at the office. Also, watch the caffeine content in beverages such as tea and soda and in pain medications—

caffeine is found in some compounds also containing aspirin and acetaminophen.

Sleep changes. Whether you snooze more or less on weekends, deviating from your typical schedule can bring on a headache. Even an hour more or less of sleep can trigger pain, says Dr. Kaiser.

Weekend eating and drinking patterns. Having a drink on the weekend to wind down can backfire: Even one drink can jump-start a headache in some people. So it's important to know your tolerance level. Sensitivities in some people to certain foods or additives, most commonly red wine and monosodium glutamate, can also trigger pain. Other foods that may trigger headaches are aged cheeses, salami and sausage.

Weekend tension. Just because it's a weekend doesn't mean you can't get stressed. In fact, stress at home can equal or even exceed pressure at the office, so monitor your general level of stress throughout the week.

Bacterial Invader
New Allergy Culprit

*I*f you have allergies, here's a strange possibility to ponder: Maybe you can control your symptoms through your stomach. Early research suggests that bacteria in the gut—the kind responsible for some peptic ulcers—may turn out to be what some allergy sufferers are sneezing at.

Out of 272 patients at an allergy clinic, 117 had been exposed to this bacteria, called *Helicobacter pylori*. Blood tests showed that about 25 percent of the people with it were allergic to it—their bodies had made allergy antibodies to this invader.

This is the first time scientists have suggested that it's possible to be allergic to bacteria. "This is exciting news because this could go a long way toward helping people with allergies be accurately diagnosed," says study leader Steven L. Kagen, M.D., assistant clinical professor of allergy and immunology at the Medical College of Wisconsin in Milwaukee.

If future studies concur, it could mean that getting the bacteria out (usually with a course of antibiotics) could take allergy symptoms with it—something that's already started to show up in clinical evidence, according to Dr. Kagen.

Dr. Kagen and his team suspected a connection between allergy and *H. pylori* when they read that ulcer medications might not work as scientists thought they did. Instead of inhibiting the acid-producing cells from releasing acid, the drugs are thought to control the inflammation that produces the acid. So, Dr. Kagen thought, the body is reacting to this invader (*H. pylori*) in a way that sounds a lot like an allergy. Coupled with the clinical knowledge that asthma often doesn't quiet down until the stomach does, Dr. Kagen tried to confirm the hypothesis in his study.

"The allergic patient requires minute amounts of exposure to get big-time symptoms," says Dr. Kagen. So the breath test for *H. pylori* might not tell you enough. If you have hives, sinus headaches or asthma, plus a busy stomach, he says, you might need to consult your physician about the possibility of having allergy antibodies to this bacteria. Presently the antibody tests are available only at Dr. Kagen's allergy clinic in Appleton, Wisconsin, but your doctor can call or write to the clinic to order these tests.

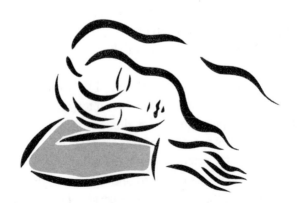

Eating Fish Builds Healthier Babies

*W*ant to build a longer, heavier baby? Try adding an extra portion of fish to your weekly diet.

Researchers compared the sizes of 1,022 babies born in the Faeroe Islands (north of the United Kingdom) with the fish-eating habits of their mothers. The more frequently the moms ate fish—up to three times a week—the larger and longer the babies were likely to be. Average increases were nearly a half-pound in weight and a centimeter in length.

Researchers speculate that the oils in fish, called omega-3 fatty acids, may facilitate blood flow (and nutrients) to the placenta. It's also possible, they say, that the oils may discourage production of the compounds that help initiate labor, so delivery doesn't happen before its time.

"Eating fish may benefit the mother as well as the fetus," says fish-oil researcher Yuping Wang, M.D., Ph.D., a research associate in the department of obstetrics and gynecology at the Medical College of Virginia in Richmond. It may also decrease the risk of preeclampsia (dangerously high blood pressure during pregnancy), she says.

If you are going to eat more fish, try those richest in omega-3 fatty acids, such as salmon, tuna and halibut. Remember that this study was about fish, not fish-oil supplements, which may not be appropriate for pregnant women. (Check with your doctor before taking any supplements during pregnancy.)

Self-Care Beats the Yeast Beast

*I*f you think you have a yeast infection, how do you decide whether to treat it yourself with an over-the-counter medication or to see a doctor for a prescription? This three-step assessment can be your guide.

1. What are your symptoms?
   a) If you have a cottage-cheese-like discharge, itching, redness, irritation or burning, go to question 2.
   b) If you have a foul-smelling discharge, fever, frequent or painful urination, or pain in the back, abdomen or shoulder, consult your doctor.
2. What's your health history?
   a) Are you pregnant?
   If no, go to 2b.
   If yes, consult your doctor.
   b) Is this your first yeast infection?
   If no, go to 2c.
   If yes, consult your doctor.
   c) How often do you get yeast infections?
   If you get fewer than two or three per year, an over-the-counter antifungal medication is a good option. Go to question 3.
   If you get more than three per year or have a recurrence within two weeks of treatment with an over-the-counter antifungal medication, consult your doctor. You may need further tests or prescription medication.
3. What form of antifungal medication is best?
   a) Do you have external irritation?
   If no, go to 3b.
   If yes, try a combination pack (suppositories plus cream to soothe external symptoms).
   b) Do you have vaginal dryness?
   If no, buy the medication you've previously used or prefer.
   If yes, try the cream formulation.

Drugs Can Trigger Sex Woes

*M*any commonly prescribed drugs can interfere with sexual function, but these negative side effects are rarely publicized. What's more, most reports in the medical literature focus on men, although women are more likely than men to be prescribed tranquilizers, antidepressants and appetite suppressants—all potentially troublesome.

Here's a sampler of prescription medications that can affect your love life. Be aware that these drugs often impede sexual function in only a small number of patients, however, and that problems related to drugs may not appear immediately. If you or your partner is experiencing any of the sexual problems listed below, ask your physician whether a drug might be the culprit and, if so, what your options are for reducing dosage or changing medications.

Drug: Tranquilizer, anti-anxiety
Brand: Valium, Xanax, Ativan
Potential Problems: Changes in libido, erection problems, delayed orgasm or ejaculation

Drug: Antidepressant
Brand: Prozac, Zoloft, Paxil, Effexor
Potential Problems: Changes in libido, delayed orgasm or ejaculation

Drug: Ulcer medication
Brand: Tagamet
Potential Problems: Decreased libido, impotence

Drug: Some birth control pills
Brand: Ortho-Novum, Loestrin, Ovcon 35 and 50 (among others)
Potential Problems: Changes in lubrication

Drug: Appetite suppressant
Brand: Pondimin
Potential Problems: Loss of libido with high doses or long-term use

Secret Signals May Hint at Bone Loss

*C*heck your mirror. Check your calendar. They may be telling you that your bones are pulling a disappearing act that could lead to disabling fractures later.

Two recent studies suggest that prematurely gray hair and irregular menstrual cycles may be secret signals of osteoporosis. But at least they signal while there's still time to take action against the problem.

Graying is called premature when half of the hair is changed by age 40. Researchers suspect that the genes that control early graying are the same as, or are very close to, those that control bone density. When scientists at the Maine Center for Osteoporosis Research, in Bangor, scanned the bones and gray hair histories of 63 people, they found that those who went prematurely gray naturally (not from another disease) had four times the chance of low bone densities than did people whose locks hadn't lost their hue.

Other clues in science suggest a bone loss/gray hair connection, too. "The most common associations with premature gray hair are thyroid disease and premature menopause. Both are associated with bone loss," says study leader Clifford Rosen, M.D., director of the Maine Center, who presented this study. Right now, there's no evidence that people who gray later in life have increased risk of low bone densities. "If you're 50 now and went gray by 40, it might be worth getting a bone-density scan to find out what your bone mass is," says Dr. Rosen. (To get information that can help de-mystify these tests, write to the National Osteoporosis Foundation, P.O. Box 96173, Department BDT, Washington, DC 20077.)

The other signal that your bones may be suffering is an irregular menstrual cycle. "Some 35-year-old women who have had irregular cycles most of their lives have bone densities that are equivalent to those of 50- or 60-year-old women," says Jerilynn C. Prior, M.D., professor of endocrinology at the University of British Columbia in Vancouver. Irregular means that cycles are too long or too short. But periods are also likely to be abnormal if they give you absolutely no clues that they're coming (a hint that you're not ovulating, even though your cycles seem regular).

The most common problem when cycles aren't normal is a lack of progesterone, suggests Dr. Prior. And when she and her research team gave that hormone for ten days a month plus one gram of calcium daily to 61 women with menstrual cycle disturbances, their bone densities increased by 2 percent. Fourteen women (with cycle disturbances) on placebo pills lost 2 percent of their bone density during the year of the study—that's the kind of loss usually seen in women only after menopause. Other calculations from the study suggest it's both the calcium and the progesterone that are helping here. There's no evidence that oral contraceptives would prevent bone loss.

"One of the things we couldn't answer before was whether a healthy premenopausal woman who has lots of calcium, who exercises regularly and who has normal weight could lose bone if she has a mixed-up period. And she can. This confirms that 'menopausal osteoporosis' can begin long before menopause," says Dr. Prior.

Other studies suggest there's still an important place for other osteoporosis prevention and treatment strategies. But if progesterone pans out in future research, says Dr. Prior, it may be an important part of the treatment of this debilitating disease.

Sweating Slowly Burns More Fat

To get the most from your stair-climber workout, don't step up your pace—slow it down! According to a recent study, those fast, short steps might not get you as far as slow, long ones if you're looking to strengthen your cardiovascular system and burn fat.

In this study, 18 people switched from quick steps that were five inches deep to slower ones that reached ten inches down from the top of the step. Energy output was about 5 percent greater with the longer step. In each test, study participants stepped for 20 minutes.

"With a smaller step, you're primarily using the smaller muscle groups," says Nicole B. Gegel, wellness consultant at Illinois State University Wellness Program in Normal, who co-authored the study with Dale D. Brown, Ph.D., assistant professor of health, physical education, recreation and dance at the university. "When larger muscle groups are recruited, you get more blood and more oxygen through the body, which benefits you by helping the heart beat faster and eventually stronger," she says.

Of course, you don't have to measure the step depth and keep vigilant over it with a video camera, as they did in the study. Just slow down enough to lengthen it a little. (The people in the study cut their number of steps almost in half.) Eight inches, the typical depth of steps in buildings, is comfortable for most people.

A few caveats: Don't work out on your toes. That's tough on the calves and can give the larger muscle groups too much of a break. Give the handrails a rest, too. Leaning may zap some of the benefits you're sweating for in the first place.

Going the Distance a Great Workout

If you hate working up a sweat and you have the time, long, slow distance walking (LSD) is a great way to work out and burn calories. Not that you'll necessarily burn more fat this way than if you do short, faster walks: That notion's becoming outdated. But you'll burn approximately as many calories as someone going at a faster pace, as long as you cover the same distance. And you're much less likely to get injured or strained.

LSD walking means putting aside 45 minutes to one hour, five to seven days a week. But don't plan a long route your first day out! If you've been inactive, start with as little as 5 to 10 minutes a day and work your way slowly to the 45- to 60-minute goal. That might take as long as three months.

Eventually, you'll need to plan one or more routes that are three to four miles long. For a while, you may want to use a route that never goes too far from home, so you can drop out and go back if you get too tired. Always keep your pace moderate so you can go the distance without pooping out.

Ten-Minute Stroll Boosts a Blue Mood

*Y*ou took the day off to let the cable-service people into the house, and they didn't get there until 3:00 P.M. The kids came home arguing, and your spouse complained about the onions in the stir-fry.

Before telling them all to take a hike, try it yourself. A few quick trips from basement to attic and back again may be all you need to undo your bad mood. Put some tunes on and you may even forget you were ever grouchy.

A survey of 308 men and women found that exercising and listening to music were the most successful ways for them to wipe out a bad mood. When 26 psychotherapists rated the smartest mood

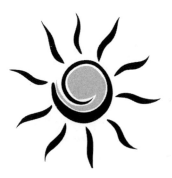

enhancers, they agreed that strategies including moving and music were winners.

You don't have to work out for days before exercise makes you feel good, either, says Robert E. Thayer, Ph.D., study author and professor of psychology at California State University, Long Beach. Walking offers immediate gratification when your mood needs a lift. A previous study by his research team found that a brisk 10-minute walk elevated energy and reduced tension (traits associated with being in a good mood) immediately, and kept doing so for at least 60 minutes.

If incessant phone calls have you glued to your desk, use your mind for a getaway. "One of the strategies that also rated very high was 'controlling thoughts.' It's kind of a potpourri of things like thinking positively, concentrating on something else and giving yourself a pep talk," says Dr. Thayer. Talking to friends or indulging in an activity you enjoy also helps move out a bad mood.

What *not* to do: happy hour (alcohol and drugs are lousy strategies). Caffeine, sweets or TV won't budge a bad mood, either. And, of course, we're talking about just negative moods, not chronic depression, which requires medical attention.

New Technology Helps Avert Surgery

One day you might not need a biopsy to know that you can relax about a suspicious spot on a mammogram. An injection of a tracer that "lights up" and a camera that's already in most hospital radiology departments may point out what's cancer and what's not without taking any tissue from the breast.

If the tracer technology, called scintimammography, is as accurate in diagnosing cancers as early reports suggest, "we can definitely have some impact on reducing the number of unnecessary biopsies," says study leader Iraj Khalkhali, M.D., chief of breast imaging at Harbor-University of California, Los Angeles Medical Center. Currently, out of every four or five biopsied tissues, only one is cancerous.

Sleuthing out breast cancers in this way is a potential new use for a technique that currently helps diagnose heart disease. Doctors don't see the technique replacing biopsy but see it as a way to narrow the pool of people who need biopsies. It could be especially useful for women with dense breasts (about 30 percent of women who get mammograms) or women whose mammograms are a tough read. A recent check of the accuracy of scintimammography matched its findings in 147 women with the biopsy results of the same women.

The technique correctly identified cancers more than 90 percent of the time (11 masses were falsely diagnosed as cancerous, while 4 were falsely diagnosed as noncancerous).

Before scintimammography becomes standard, doctors are awaiting the results of large clinical trials. For now, says Dr. Khalkhali, "we recommend that every woman go for a biopsy if her doctor recommends it. We don't want any cancer missed."

Regular Workouts Protect Breasts

*W*hat's ten minutes out of the morning? Thirty more after work? In the amount of time it takes the coffee to brew and the dinner to bake, you could go a long way toward knocking down your breast cancer risk.

About four hours of exercise a week may reduce the risk of premenopausal breast cancer by an average of 58 percent, according to a recent study. Researchers compared the lifetime exercise habits of 545 premenopausal women who had breast cancer with 545 premenopausal but cancer-free women. Benefits were even greater for the most active exercisers with children: Their risk was reduced by 72 percent, compared with a 27 percent reduction in risk for exercisers without kids.

This cancer's not like lung cancer, where the major risk factor is a controllable one (smoking). Pregnancies, family history, age of menstruation onset and socioeconomic status are factors that seem to have some play in determining breast cancer risk. And right now, the effects of diet on breast cancer are still controversial, says study leader Leslie Bernstein, Ph.D., professor of preventive medicine at the University of Southern California School of Medicine, Los Angeles. So the idea that exercise may lower risk significantly (if this study is confirmed by future ones)—and that it's something you can take control of—provides some hope to women seeking anything to help stem the epidemic.

The going theory is that exercise diminishes the breast's exposure to hormones by changing the length of the menstrual cycle or by helping to smooth out its hormonal peaks, says Dr. Bernstein.

"Probably the most important finding was that lifetime patterns of exercise appeared to be important," she says. Those who accrued more hours of exercise—people who started exercising in their teens or early twenties—reduced their risks most significantly. But even women who began substantial exercise programs later were protected.

The group with reduced risk in this study engaged in a spectrum of activities—jogging, racquet sports, swimming, strenuous walking and weight lifting. So researchers can't yet say whether the biggest benefits might come from resistance training or aerobic training. The bottom line for now is to get moving.

"We already know that you ought to maintain a regular exercise program, based on the reduction in risk of heart disease, adult-onset diabetes, osteoporosis and colon cancer," says Dr. Bernstein. "The possible reduction in breast cancer risk just adds greater fuel to that."

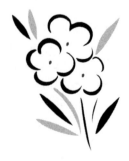

If the evidence makes you want to renew your health club membership, researchers encourage you to make it a family pass. A big implication of this study is for children, Dr. Bernstein says. "People who research breast cancer are concerned that young people aren't being introduced to regular exercise habits." But by making exercise a part of their lifestyles, they'll have a habit that may have major health benefits in adulthood.

Retin-A May Zap Precancerous Growth

Smoothing wrinkles and zapping acne may be only part of the power of Retin-A. Research hints that this vitamin-A-derived drug may knock out cervical cancer before it can get a firm start.

Researchers tested a cream containing all-trans-retinoic acid (Retin-A) against a dummy cream in more than 200 women with moderate or severe precancerous changes. Women used the cream for a total of eight days throughout the six months of the study. In women with moderate dysplasia, the precancerous cells completely regressed in 43 percent of the treatment group, compared to 27 percent of women using dummy cream.

"If this works, it could be a simpler and less invasive way of treating this problem," says Stephen C. Rubin, M.D., director of gynecological oncology at the University of Pennsylvania Medical Center in Philadelphia. The idea is that you'd get a prescription, rather than laser surgery, to zap these cells gone awry.

What's more, researchers see the implications of this study going far beyond the cervix. "It's only the third big trial to show that it may be possible to reverse or suppress cancer at an early stage," says study leader Frank L. Meyskens, Jr., M.D., director of the University of California, Irvine, Cancer Center.

The fact that there were no benefits for women with severe dysplasia could suggest that as cells get further along in their changes, they get less responsive. That's a good reason for getting regular Pap smears.

Researchers aren't yet sure of the mechanisms by which Retin-A could be helping cells get healthy. But they suspect it may slow the growth of these cervical cells that have put proliferation in overdrive.

"Right now, it remains to be seen how this cream will actually be used when it gets out of the experimental stage," says Dr. Meyskens. "But this belongs to the first generation of important papers in the area of therapies that alter the natural history of cancer."

Low-Fat Diet Curtails Cancer Threat

*U*sed to be you had to have a child or actively prevent one with oral contraceptives to lower your risk of ovarian cancer. But recent research shifts the focus from the kids to the kitchen. Findings suggest that ovarian cancer may also be thwarted with foods like sugar snap peas and skim milk.

When researchers evaluated the eating habits of 450 women with ovarian cancer and 564 without, they saw that cutting ten grams of saturated fat a day (that's a switch from two glasses of whole milk to

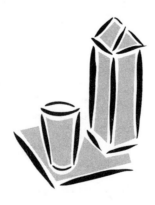

the same amount of skim) could trim the risk of ovarian cancer by 20 percent. And adding ten grams of vegetable fiber—what you'd find in about one cup of cooked lentils—may take down the risk another 37 percent. The study saw no relationship between unsaturated fats and risks for this cancer.

Small studies have hinted at links between diet and reduced risk of ovarian cancer, but this first, large study of the issues gives the idea some real weight.

"It appears possible to cut your risk of ovarian cancer in half by an aggressive modification of the diet," says Harvey A. Risch, M.D., Ph.D., associate professor of epidemiology and public health at Yale University School of Medicine.

Theories abound about how diet might affect hormones. Meat and dairy foods may contain small amounts of estrogen. Estrogen-like compounds are also found in vegetables. The brain may think they're the real hormone and halt its own production. Or the fiber in those vegetables may grab estrogen and escort it out of the body.

Of course, the diet this study points toward isn't all that Spartan. Studies suggest most people eat more saturated fat than they need to, and cutting it by a third by switching protein sources much of the time is a smart thing to do for other health benefits, too.

"The point isn't that people should never eat hamburgers," he says. "But things that are eaten regularly that are high in saturated fat should be cut back. People don't realize how little meat protein they need per day to live perfectly well. Four ounces of meat a day is probably sufficient for most women."

Video Quells "Dental Dread"

*I*f you dread going to the dentist, you may need glasses—video glasses, that is.

These wraparound glasses create a personal cinema by projecting a video image on the glasses. Once the eyewear's built-in headphones are placed in your ears, the system shuts out the sight and sound of the drill.

For years, dentists have tried to calm nervous patients through relaxation techniques. A favorite is guided imagery, when you may be asked to imagine yourself on a beach. "Now, with this technology, we can actually show you the beach and let you hear the surf," says Frank Grimaldi, D.D.S., assistant clinical professor and director of hospital dentistry at the University of California, San Francisco.

Select a VCR video from your dentist's collection, bring your own or get the device hooked up for cable viewing. The point is to sit back, relax and feel comfortable while your mouth is open wide. Just don't expect any popcorn.

To receive a list of the dentists in your area who are currently using the eyewear, contact Micro-Vac at 1-800-729-1020.

PART TWO

Staying Well

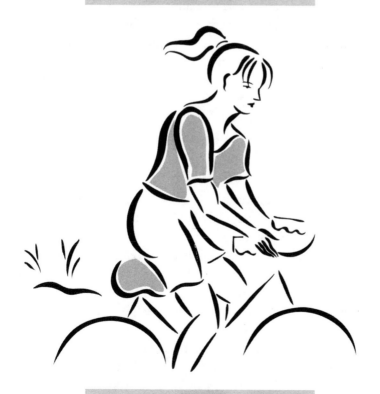

Decoding Your Body's Distress Signals

Learning to read and act on these red alerts can help protect and save you from a variety of illnesses.

Among her many patients, Atlanta physician Joy Church, M.D., recalls two in particular. "One woman came in once a month and complained each time of something she swore was life threatening," says Dr. Church. "If she had a cough, she thought it was pneumonia. If she had a mole, she was sure it was skin cancer." She was usually in perfect health.

"The other patient was brought into my office by her family for a problem with her breast," says Dr. Church. "She kept saying, 'It's nothing—really, it's nothing.' But her breast was badly diseased. She said it was just an infection and that she was washing it with alcohol." Shortly after being admitted to the hospital, this woman died of breast cancer.

While these patients and their problems appear very different, they are in essence the same: Neither woman was able to correctly interpret the signals her body was sending her. In other words, neither woman understood how to read her body.

Learning "Symptomspeak"

While the notion of "reading your body" (also known as symptomspeak) may sound annoyingly New Age, it's really a rather basic but scientifically sound concept.

Symptomspeak is your body's bridge between the physical and the psychological. It's a kind of mental Morse code that transmits various subtle, and sometimes not so subtle, signals that your body sends out, from an abdominal ache to a bloody stool. Deciphering this code is the best and most efficient way to keep tabs on your health and protect yourself from the advancement of a variety of illnesses.

Consider breast cancer, for instance. Ninety-three percent of women who find and seek treatment for breast cancer early, before it has spread beyond the breast, will survive. If they're diagnosed after it has progressed, however, their odds of survival drop dramatically.

The same is true of heart disease, the number one killer of women. "Yet if a woman has a pain in the upper left portion of her body, she assumes it's a pulled muscle," says Felicia Stewart, M.D., director of research for Sumter Medical Foundation in Sacramento, California, and author of Understanding Your Body: Every Woman's Guide to Gynecology and Health. "Since many people still view heart disease as a male condition, women don't recognize the signs of heart disease." They misread—or fail to read—their body's signals.

Conditions less dire than breast cancer or heart disease may also require medical attention. And in many cases, your doctor can tell you how to relieve your pain and to prevent a more serious problem from developing later on.

Of course, as Dr. Church's anecdote about her overanxious patient illustrates, not all bodily signs require immediate attention. Somewhere between the extremes represented by Dr. Church's two patients lies the ability to hear and understand your body's language—to know when a symptom needs medical attention and when it doesn't.

Most experts believe that women read their bodies fairly well—at least compared to men. "Because of changes in our reproductive systems, more things happen on a regular basis in women's bodies than in men's," says Rita Charon, M.D., associate professor of clinical medicine at the College of Physicians and Surgeons of Columbia University in New York City. "As a result, we become accustomed to change and its signs."

But recognizing a symptom or two is only half the battle. You also have to interpret the problem *and* decide what to do about it. Following are four common symptoms, a discussion of possible causes and a primer on how to read them.

Abdominal Pain: Many Causes, Many Cures

"I have a stomachache" is a catchall complaint we've all used to describe pain throughout the midsection. Your mission is to pinpoint the true cause of the trouble so you can treat your pain effectively.

Dining on spicy foods, succumbing to a viral infection or over-indulging in food or drink can cause gastritis, an inflammation of the lining of the stomach, which is located in the upper part of the midsection just below the rib cage. Gastritis is a true "stomachache" and is often accompanied by nausea and vomiting. Going without food for four to six hours, then eating only bland foods such as toast and crackers and sipping ginger ale or another clear liquid for four to six hours often provides relief. Antacids and over-the-counter medications such as Pepto-Bismol also may do the trick.

Another common source of stomach pain is the ulcer, an inflammation of the lining of the stomach often brought on by bacteria, smoking, stress, alcohol, caffeine or aspirin. In some people, these habits, products and conditions produce acids that eat away at the stomach lining and create a burning feeling just below the breastbone that's especially pronounced when the stomach is empty. Steering clear of preventable triggers and gulping products such as Maalox may dull the discomfort. But treating yourself is generally a bad idea. If you experience ulcerlike symptoms, see your physician. She may prescribe medication for your condition.

A third source of stomach distress is constipation (going three or more days without a bowel movement), which can cause bouts of cramping, gas, bloating and pain in the lower abdomen. Possible culprits include inadequate fiber and fluid intake or insufficient exercise. A big bowl of bran cereal should be your first pain prescription. If that doesn't work, then reach for a liquid laxative. If your constipation persists, consult your physician. You might ask her about starting a regular weight-bearing exercise routine and a fiber-rich diet, both of which will help get your digestive system back on track.

Menstrual cramps are a uniquely feminine brand of tummy trouble. Caused by hormonelike chemicals called prostaglandins that are released in the body during menstruation, normal period pain is easy to pinpoint (because it coincides with your cycle). It's also simple to treat with nonsteroidal anti-inflammatory drugs such as ibuprofen or the prescription drug Anaprox.

If your pain is disabling or accompanied by other symptoms such as bleeding between periods, heavier than normal bleeding or pain during intercourse, something serious could be the culprit. Pain associated with endometriosis (a condition that results when pieces of the uterine lining break away and implant in the lower abdomen) or fibroid tumors (nonmalignant growths in the uterus) is often confused with "normal" menstrual pain—but it's far from normal. While both conditions can be treated with drugs or surgery, they must be caught early: If left untreated, these conditions can cause dire problems such as infertility.

If you experience any of the symptoms above, or any of the following symptoms, see your doctor immediately.

- Pain or cramps after meals, which can signal a hiatal hernia
- Pain that is sharp, severe or localized—a symptom of appendicitis
- Chronic cramps, which could point to irritable bowel syndrome or other serious digestive disorders
- Pain that is accompanied by a fever, vomiting or other severe symptoms
- Discomfort accompanied by extreme bloating, which could signal the presence of a growth, such as a tumor

Headache: Not Always Stress-Induced

The pounding is excruciating, the pain persistent. This is no garden-variety headache, you tell yourself. This must be something more.

Don't be so sure. The National Headache Foundation estimates that every year, 45 million Americans suffer from standard head pain severe enough to cause them to miss work or visit a doctor. Just about anything can spark a head splitter—missing your morning coffee, stress, muscle tension, colds and the flu, low blood sugar, allergies and fatigue. And just about all headaches can be eased by reducing stress, exercising, stretching tight muscles, draining your sinuses with medication, eating small meals throughout the day, taking pain relievers or massaging your head and scalp.

Not so with migraines, which are characterized by severe, throbbing pain restricted to one side of the head and often accompanied by nausea and sensitivity to light and other stimuli. About 10 to 15 percent of people—mainly women—suffer from migraines, which tend to run in families. Menstruation, birth control pills, some foods such as chocolate, cheese and monosodium glutamate, poor air quality and stressful situations bring them on. While some women find relief by lying quietly in a dark room, using an ice pack to constrict blood vessels in the head and taking ibuprofen (such as Advil or Nuprin) or aspirin (such as Excedrin), others require prescription medication.

A headache is very rarely the sign of a serious neurological disorder. But if you have a headache coupled with any of the following symptoms or scenarios, seek medical help immediately.

- Eye pain or double or blurred vision
- A severe head injury
- Weakness or loss of feeling in any part of the body
- Nausea, vomiting or convulsions
- A blackout or fainting spell

Chest Pain: Don't Panic

You've just come from Sunday dinner at your mother-in-law's house and a piano has settled atop your chest. That dear woman's sarcasm and your husband's nonchalance may have sent you into cardiac arrest—but probably not.

Rather, your mother-in-law's fat-laden food most likely has triggered gastroesophageal reflux—better known as heartburn—which occurs when stomach acids creep up and burn the esophagus, the tube that connects the throat to the stomach. Heartburn can arise if you've eaten spicy foods or overindulged, drunk alcohol or coffee or taken aspirin or other medications.

To relieve (and avoid) this bothersome chest pain, steer clear of these triggers. Also, try elevating the head of your bed four to six inches from the ground (with blocks or books) to prevent food and acids from sneaking up into your esophagus. (Using pillows under your head won't do the trick.) You can also take antacids after eating—just be sure to sit up rather than lie down after taking the medication. If your heartburn refuses to dissipate, consult your physician.

NINE SIGNALS YOU SHOULDN'T IGNORE

Some body signals are serious. See a doctor if you experience the following:

- Abnormal menstrual bleeding (Watch for a sudden, heavy period or bleeding between periods or after sex.)
- Frequent, painful or bloody urination
- Blood in your stool
- Any growth or mass
- A severe, persistent headache accompanied by eye pain, double or blurred vision, weakness or numbness in any part of the body, nausea, vomiting, convulsions or fainting
- Dizziness, fainting or sudden changes in vision

- Fever that lasts for more than 24 hours and doesn't respond to acetaminophen or aspirin and is not associated with a common virus (or any fever above 104°F)
- Vomiting or diarrhea that lasts for more than 48 hours and doesn't respond to changes in diet or over-the-counter medication
- Chest pain with a sensation of pressure, fullness, squeezing or pain in the center of the chest that lasts for more than a few minutes or subsides and then returns

Panic disorder, a condition often confused with a heart attack, is another common cause of chest pain. More than three million Americans suffer from panic disorder, which usually involves short, unpredictable attacks of intense fear accompanied by chest pain, shortness of breath, heart palpitations, dizziness and sweating. Although its symptoms are similar to those of a heart attack, a panic attack is also accompanied by an intense emotional response—usually overwhelming fear and powerlessness. And panic attacks tend to strike young women, but heart attack victims are generally middle-age or older. If you suspect you're suffering from panic disorder, talk to your doctor. She most likely will give you a physical exam to rule out heart problems and may want you to go to a psychiatrist, who can prescribe coping techniques and medication if the problem persists.

Chest pain *can* also signal a heart attack. But too many women

BREAST LUMP? DON'T PANIC

*I*t's that time of the month and your breasts are tender. Wait— make that painful. With lumps. Should you worry?

Chances are, no. While it's always smart to consult your doctor about any changes you notice in your breasts, in nine out of ten cases, breast lumps are harmless. The common culprit? Fibrocystic disease, a benign condition in which fluid-filled cysts cause breast pain. The remedy? Certain lifestyle changes, like avoiding caffeine and fatty foods and quitting smoking.

Some symptoms warrant a doctor's visit, though. They are:

• A firm, irregular, immobile lump
• Puckered or dimpled skin over the lump
• Any nipple changes, such as bleeding
• Swollen glands in the armpit
• Pain around the lump area

dismiss this possibility because they consider cardiovascular problems "a man's disease"—and they couldn't be more wrong.

Pay special attention to chest pain if you're at risk for developing heart disease. The risk factors include a family history of the disease, increasing age, smoking, high blood pressure, high cholesterol, physical inactivity and obesity. And learn the warning signs for a heart attack, which include uncomfortable pressure, fullness, squeezing or pain in the center of the chest; pain spreading from the chest to the shoulders, neck or arms; and lightheadedness, fainting, sweating, nausea or shortness of breath. If you experience any of these symptoms, seek medical help immediately.

Fatigue: Help for Chronic Tiredness

Fatigue is a funny thing. Sometimes it's a symptom—the body's way of fighting off a virus or infection—and sometimes the ailment itself. Sometimes fatigue is fueled by not-so-serious factors such as stress, premenstrual syndrome, poor eating habits, lack of exercise or boredom; other times, it's stoked by serious conditions such as cancer or depression. And sometimes it's chronic fatigue syndrome (CFS).

People with CFS feel achy, feverish and exhausted all the time for no apparent reason. Their symptoms may begin with an illness such as bronchitis, hepatitis or the flu, or they may surface gradually, occur out of the blue or afflict someone who is highly stressed.

Experts believe CFS is caused by a virus or a breakdown of the immune system, and CFS has been linked with herpes, candidiasis, environmental illness and HIV. Fatigue is also often confused with Lyme disease and multiple sclerosis. But no one knows for sure why it strikes—and no one has discovered a cure. Doctors simply treat the symptoms—usually through diet, light exercise and other lifestyle changes that help reduce stress.

To determine the origin of prolonged fatigue, Dr. Charon suggests taking stock of everything (other than fatigue) that is bothering you— from a stressful job or family situation to your diet. Then tackle those problems and see how you feel. If you remain fatigued, consult your physician. If you think your fatigue may be linked to an emotional concern, consider seeking counseling or joining a support group.

Peri-What?

You're having hot flashes and periods. What gives?
These strategies can help you handle perimenopause.

Just after her 40th birthday, Maria Lewis began to experience painful midcycle cramping. Then the ache in her belly seemed to shatter and spread. And over the next three years, she suffered intermittent heart palpitations, weight gain, achy joints, sleep disturbances, increased premenstrual jitteriness, short-term memory loss, free-floating anxiety (anxiety with no known trigger) and frequent "blushing"—all for no reason she could fathom. Convinced she was either approaching menopause or crazy, Lewis sought the help of her gynecologist. "I was having hot flashes and regular periods," she says.

"Yet my doctor dismissed menopause as improbable. She said I was far too young."

Lewis wasn't so sure. So she did a little digging on her own—and hit pay dirt in the form of Janine O'Leary Cobb's *Understanding Menopause*. While paging though the book, Lewis happened upon a list of perimenopausal ailments Cobb had culled from letters written to her over the past decade by the 17,000 women who have subscribed to her newsletter, *A Friend Indeed*. All of Lewis's symptoms were on it.

"I read through the list and thought, 'Wow, this is me—I'm perfectly normal.' And I felt immediate relief," she says. "It made me realize that what doctors call menopause and what women experience as menopause aren't always one and the same."

Not by a long shot. What Lewis was experiencing wasn't menopause as doctors define it—a single event that marks the end of a woman's monthly periods and reproductive life. It was what one menopause expert refers to as "the changes before the change"—or, in technical jargon, the "climacteric."

During this stage, which is thought to commence at about age 35, your periods may flow like clockwork and you may be 15 years from full-fledged menopause, but your ovaries begin to run out of the half million or so eggs you were born with and the levels of estrogen and progesterone in your body start to drop. The first noticeable indication? Often, it's infertility. But there may be other signs as well, as Maria Lewis discovered.

More Than Just Hot Flashes

Given that the climacteric has occurred since the dawn of time, it's surprising how little is actually known about it. "Indeed, we know more about the natural history of AIDS than we do about a woman's transition to menopause," says Jerilynn C. Prior, M.D., associate professor of medicine at the University of British Columbia in Vancouver.

Consequently, doctors may not associate achy joints, heart palpitations, free-floating anxiety and other ailments with menopause—primarily because this clutch of symptoms doesn't support the accepted medical model: that menopause equals estrogen deprivation. "In fact, I find that many doctors are locked into the mindset that if a condition isn't alleviated by estrogen, it can't have anything to do with menopause," says Cobb, a nationally recognized expert on menopause.

Dr. Prior concurs. When she lectures to doctors, she routinely asks them how they would treat a woman in her mid-forties who suffers from frequent migraines, weight gain, breast swelling and night sweats. Some of these symptoms are the hallmark of high estrogen and some are associated with low estrogen; all are reported by women approaching menopause.

"The responses I receive are pretty incredible," says Dr. Prior, whose hypothetical patient suffers from some of the symptoms she herself is now experiencing as part of the climacteric. "Most physicians say they would refer the patient to a counselor for emotional support, offer her a sedative or check her thyroid. In other words, most would assume that her problems are all imagined."

They're not. Symptoms commonly associated with the climacteric, such as joint pain, sleep disturbances, memory loss, discomfort during sex, stress incontinence and free-floating anxiety, have their basis in biology, not psychology. And all of them can be alleviated, often with simple measures. Here's what some of the menopause experts (if not the M.D.'s) recommend.

Vitamins for Joint Pain

While the hot flash is the symptom most people—women and doctors included—associate with menopause, studies show that joint pain not associated with arthritis is the problem many menopausal women suffer from most.

What causes this pain? No one knows for sure. But Cobb suspects that the climacteric affects the adrenal glands, where the precursor to estrone (a substance that's changed into a form of estrogen in the body) and cortisone (which keeps your joints lubricated) are produced.

She recommends that women plagued by joint pain first be tested for arthritis. Once that's ruled out, she suggests visiting a physical therapist—and experimenting with vitamins. Some of the women who write to her say they've found relief by taking a daily combination of vitamin E (400 international units), cod liver oil (one capsule or one teaspoon) and vitamin B_6 (1.5 to 2 milligrams daily), which doctors sometimes prescribe to relieve symptoms of carpal tunnel syndrome (numbness, tingling and pain in the thumb, index and middle fingers).

Stay Cool and Sleep Better

Many women approaching menopause suffer from a particular kind of insomnia: They may fall asleep before their heads hit the pillow, but a few hours later they wake up suddenly with a rapid heartbeat or an urge to toss off the covers.

"They're experiencing a subtle form of the hot flash," explains Judith Seifer, R.N., Ph.D., a West Virginia sex therapist who lectures women's and physician's groups on the climacteric. "This isn't a full-blown hot flash or night sweats but a blushing or warm sensation that's caused by the same trigger—fluctuations in estrogen levels.

"These heat fluctuations may occur during the daytime, too—which may explain Lewis's frequent 'blushing.' But they tend to be less obvious then, because you are usually more distracted," says Dr. Seifer. "You may notice a little dampness under your bra, or think, 'Oh no, my deodorant's failing.' But that's about it."

Nighttime body temperature changes, on the other hand, generally prove more bothersome. If you're losing sleep because of them, try exercising daily, avoiding caffeine and alcohol, drinking warm milk in the evening and indulging in a relaxation technique such as yoga before you go to bed. If these measures don't do the trick, talk with your physician about prescribing low-dose estrogen replacement therapy (ERT) or an oral contraceptive. "Most women sleep through the night after a week or two on hormone therapy," says Dr. Seifer.

You should also try to stay cool. When you experience a flush, your body temperature rises just as it does when you have a fever. So you'll stay cooler—and be less likely to wake up—if you wear cotton rather than nylon or flannel to bed. "This means no more Victoria's Secret nylon nighties," says Dr. Seifer.

Forgetful or Just Plain Busy?

Lewis had always prided herself on her keen memory. But that was before she found herself purposefully striding into rooms—and then wondering why she was there. "I can sing the entire theme song to the old TV show *Maverick*," she says. "So why can't I remember when my son needs to be picked up from soccer practice?"

Experts aren't sure—in part because they really haven't examined the phenomenon closely. Cobb says she has searched the medical literature on menopause for information on these fairly typical memory lapses but has found only a handful of relevant studies. "The research indicates that there are slight memory differences between younger women and menopausal women and between women who have lost their ovaries and those who haven't, but the differences aren't significant or lasting," she says. "In fact, the memories of all the women studied are very similar."

The problem, Cobb speculates, is that most women have overdeveloped memories—primarily because they're routinely called upon to remember things for other people: sports and activity schedules for their children, dinner dates for their husbands, doctor's appointments for their parents. "So while our memories may slip a little during menopause," she says, "they're only falling from the extraordinary to the normal."

Still, memory lapses can be confounding when they occur. So Dr. Seifer suggests making lists until the problem disappears—usually along with menopause.

The Secret to Sexual Satisfaction

Many women approaching menopause experience sexual changes, both physical and emotional, good and bad. Most are associated with the dips in estrogen that begin during the climacteric.

First, the good: "Up until age 50, your estrogen level declines but not consistently," says Dr. Seifer. "So you experience intermittent peaks and valleys of estrogen. And when your estrogen dips down low, your testosterone peaks—along with your sex drive."

Problem is, estrogen stimulates cell growth and vaginal lubrication. So its slow decline can lead to thinning of vaginal tissue and inadequate lubrication, both of which can cause irritation during intercourse. And that's not all: Because the cardiovascular and the peripheral and central nervous systems are also influenced by estrogen, women in their climacteric can experience a decline in blood flow to their genitals, a drop in physical responsiveness and a loss of sexual desire.

Still other women experience touch impairment—an aversion to being touched (sexually or nonsexually) that may be hormone-based as well. "This is often the secret symptom," Dr. Seifer says, "the one nobody ever talks about. And it's a real problem for women who've delayed childbearing. They have younger children who tend to cling to their legs, and the women can't stand it. They end up pushing their families away because they feel suffocated."

Of course, there are several steps you can take to combat the sexual changes associated with menopause. You can use a water-based lubricant such as K-Y Jelly or Replens during intercourse to combat vaginal dryness. And you can ask your doctor about prescribing low-dose ERT—specifically, a pill that contains both estrogen and androgen (the male hormone, the most active of which is testosterone). Although in some women it does produce a few unsavory side effects such as excess hair growth and deepening of the voice, these problems can usually be reversed by adjusting the dosage. And androgen boosts the sex drive of most women who take it.

You can also talk to your partner about how you feel. "Chances are, he knows something's different," says Dr. Seifer. "He just doesn't know what it is." Let him in on your feelings. Then you can work on the problem together.

Natural Help for Urine Leaks

A big word for an embarrassing problem, stress incontinence refers to the involuntary escape of small amounts of urine when you cough, laugh, exercise or lift heavy objects. The culprit? Weakened sphincter muscles surrounding the urethra. Childbearing stretches these muscles, so it's responsible for many cases of stress incontinence. But the tissues in the lower urethra and sphincter that regulate urine flow are also influenced by estrogen. And when its level in the body wanes, these tissues become weak.

A cycle of low-dose ERT can often eradicate stress incontinence, says Dr. Seifer. But nonhormonal measures can be just as effective. Ask your doctor for information on bladder training and exercises such as Kegels to strengthen the muscles in your pelvic floor. (To find out how to perform Kegels, see "How to Kegel Correctly" on page 79.)

Having sex may also help, says Dr. Prior. "The tissue surrounding the urethra is erectile tissue, similar to a man's penile tissue," she says. "So if you're feeling sexy because your hormones are high but you aren't having sex, there may be some swelling around the urethra. And incontinence can result."

Ride Out Occasional Jitters

Many women fear that depression is a natural consequence of menopause. But research simply doesn't bear this out. Fact is, women approaching menopause are more likely to suffer from anxiety, as Maria Lewis did, than depression.

Many women experience free-floating anxiety as foreboding—a sense that something is going to happen to them or to someone they love—while others may experience it as a loss of confidence. Cobb herself recalls that after years of teaching, she suddenly became very self-conscious walking into a classroom. "I just had this feeling that I was going to fall down or make a fool of myself," she says.

But anxiety can manifest itself in many ways, some of the most common being shallow breathing, a heaviness in the chest, an accelerated heart rate and an overwhelming feeling that your health and well-being are at risk. If you're experiencing any of these symptoms, consult your doctor. She will set your mind at ease about their cause (most likely, you don't have heart disease or cancer, for instance) and help you to better understand your anxiety and its various manifestations. In addition, you should consider exercising regularly, indulging in relaxation techniques and avoiding stimulants such as nicotine and caffeine.

Group therapy—formal or informal—may also make you feel better about this confusing stage, says Dr. Prior, who suggests sharing your experiences with other women about your age. "We've traditionally gone to our doctors for information that we could have gathered from our female friends, and we've come up short," she says. "Only by talking to each other will we discover that other women have endured similar experiences, that we're not crazy and that we'll survive this stage of our lives."

Making Peace with Menopause

Menopause is a process, not a disease. Here's how to cope with its symptoms and get on with your life.

Okay, so you don't want to hear about it. You don't even want to think about it. You figure you're too young for menopause. And besides, you've heard about its discomforts—hot flashes, mood swings and vaginal dryness, to name a few.

But menopause doesn't have to be terrible. In fact, when women share their experiences they often find that it doesn't have to be the beginning of old age. Instead, menopause can mark the start of a new phase in life, one that is vital, productive and fulfilling.

What to Expect from the Change

An estimated 40 to 50 million women—more than ever before—will enter menopause in the next two decades. Most American women hit menopause around age 51. Some women go through it earlier, and an estimated 1 percent do so before age 40.

Menopause begins after a woman's last period. A woman is considered to be in menopause after she hasn't menstruated for a full year. But before that happens, women go through a phase known as the climacteric, or perimenopause. At this time, the ovaries get smaller and produce less estrogen. This drop is what causes the hot flashes, night sweats, vaginal dryness, skin changes, sleep difficulties, mood swings, depression and weight gain experienced by some women. The drop in estrogen often alters a woman's period, which may become heavier or lighter, longer or shorter or irregular. And symptoms of premenstrual syndrome (PMS) can worsen.

Menopause can bring physical and emotional changes. Because of hormonal shifts, women sometimes can feel out of control. "It can be a real up-and-down time," says Joan Borton, a licensed mental health counselor in Rockport, Massachusetts, who runs workshops for menopausal women and is the author of *Drawing from the Women's Well: Reflections on the Life Passage of Menopause*. "That is very disconcerting for women, particularly those who have been able to feel like they are on top of things."

But the changes women fear do not always occur, experts say. Studies indicate that between 16 and 38 percent of menopausal women are symptom-free—no hot flashes, no dryness, no nothing.

And even if women do have symptoms, they don't happen overnight, and they don't turn women into wrinkled old ladies. On the contrary, women often feel sexy, productive, bright and relieved that they no longer need to worry about getting pregnant, says Ellen Klutznick, Psy.D., a psychotherapist in San Francisco who counsels menopausal women.

And some women truly branch out. During menopause many women evaluate what they have done, what they are doing and where they are going, says Borton. "There is a sense of excitement among many women at this time, as well as a real sense of urgency," she says. Women commonly tell her, "For this last third of my life I want to give my energy to things that are real core concerns to me. I'm not going to give my energy to peripheral stuff anymore."

The Role of HRT

But even if a woman approaches menopause with positive feelings, there are changes going on inside her body that put her at risk for certain diseases. When estrogen drops, for instance, a woman's risk of heart disease increases: Estrogen exerts a protective effect on the heart by keeping levels of "good" cholesterol, or high-density lipoprotein (HDL), high, and levels of "bad" cholesterol, or low-density lipoprotein (LDL), low.

Declining levels of estrogen also place women at increased risk for osteoporosis. This is because estrogen plays a key role in stimulating bone growth and promoting the absorption of calcium. When estrogen levels drop, these effects do too.

These disease risks and the physical changes that some women go through are why some women consider hormone replacement therapy (HRT)—therapy designed to replenish a woman's diminishing hormones.

While there are different types of HRT, most doctors recommend ones that include estrogen and a synthetic form of proges-terone called progestin. Estrogen is used for its beneficial effect on the heart and bones, among other things. But when given alone, es-trogen can stimulate cancer growth in the uterus and breast. Prog-estin cuts that risk.

Whether to take HRT is one of the biggest questions women con-front about menopause, says Borton. It is a difficult personal decision, she says, because there are pros and cons.

Among the benefits of HRT is relief from hot flashes and vaginal dryness—the two symptoms that drive most women to ask about the therapy, says Brian Walsh, M.D., director of the Menopause Clinic at Brigham and Women's Hospital in Boston.

From a health standpoint, a big plus for HRT is the protection from heart disease it provides, experts say. In studies of women who took just estrogen, doctors found that it appeared to lower women's risk of heart disease by 50 percent compared to women who didn't take it. Thorough studies on HRT—which provides both estrogen and progestin—have yet to be done, but initial research shows that HRT may also offer substantial protection against heart disease.

Hormone replacement therapy can also prevent women from de-veloping osteoporosis. Research suggests that women who take HRT reduce their risk of osteoporosis-related fractures by 50 percent, and women who have the disease may be able to increase their bone den-sity by 5 percent through HRT.

Considering HRT? Read This First

HRT is not without its risks, cautions Dr. Walsh. The greatest concern is whether taking HRT will increase the risk of uterine or breast cancer.

Of postmenopausal women not taking HRT, one in 1,000 will de-velop uterine cancer, according to studies. For women who take estro-gen alone, that risk increases between two and ten times, depending on how much estrogen is in the formulation they take and how long they take it.

Studies indicate, however, that when progestin is taken with es-trogen, the risk of uterine cancer is lower than when estrogen is taken

HRT OPTIONS: CHOOSING THE THERAPY THAT'S RIGHT FOR YOU

*N*ot all hormone replacement therapy (HRT) prescriptions are the same. There are different timetables for taking the formulations, which can come as a cream, patch or pill.

In one type of HRT, called sequential therapy, estrogen is taken every day for two weeks. Then, on the 15th day, progestin is taken as well. Both estrogen and progestin are continued from day 15 through day 25, and then both are withdrawn. It's at this time that menstrual-like bleeding begins.

In another method called continuous combined therapy, both estrogen and progestin are taken every day. This method was developed as a means to eliminate the bleeding that occurs with sequential therapy, and it's currently the most common regimen used. Initially, women on continuous combined therapy experience irregular bleeding. In time, the menstrual-like bleeding will cease, but that can take up to six months.

Estrogen creams are often used by women who experience vaginal dryness. The cream is inserted with an applicator directly into the vagina, where it works to replenish vaginal tissue. In the beginning, vaginal estrogen cream is used three to four times a week, until vaginal symptoms improve. Then it's used less frequently.

Estrogen patches are often the choice of women who want to take HRT but can't take estrogen orally because of gallbladder disease. The patch, called Estraderm, is the size of a small bandage and is worn on the lower abdomen. The estrogen is absorbed through the skin and then released directly into the bloodstream in timed sequences.

Estrogen pills are taken by mouth, according to the regimen set by your doctor. Premarin is the most commonly used pill. It's a natural form of estrogen—mare's estrogen—whereas some other estrogen pills are synthetic.

How effective HRT is in fighting heart disease depends on which type of estrogen you use, according to Brian Walsh, M.D., director of the Menopause Clinic at Brigham and Women's Hospital in Boston. Estrogen creams and the patch are not as effective as pills. With the pill, estrogen passes through the digestive tract and liver, where it exerts its impact on cholesterol. With the patch and cream, however, estrogen goes directly into the bloodstream, and the effect on cholesterol is diminished.

by itself. In a ten-year study of 398 women taking both hormones, none of the women who took progestin for at least 10 days out of 25 developed uterine cancer. Whether women who take HRT are at lower risk for uterine cancer than women who don't take any hormones has not been conclusively proven, but based on preliminary studies, doctors suspect that the risk may be lower by an estimated 30 to 40 percent.

If a woman decides to take only estrogen, she can be monitored for uterine cancer by her doctor.

Breast cancer is a concern for women on HRT. Estrogen promotes cancer growth in lab animals, so there's reason to suspect that giving women estrogen might stimulate breast cancer. While research on breast cancer risk from HRT has yielded no definite conclusion, a study conducted at the Centers for Disease Control and Prevention in Atlanta determined that a woman's risk may be relative to how long she's on the therapy. Women in the study who took hormones the longest—for more than 15 years—had the greatest risk, and it was 30 percent higher than for women who did not take HRT or took it for less than 5 years.

Women who take HRT are also at risk for gallstones, particularly during the first year of therapy, says Dr. Walsh. Also, if you've had cancer of the breast or uterus, have active liver disease or have had major problems with blood clots, HRT is not usually recommended.

A Pre-menopause "To-Do" List

Menopause may bring some physical changes, but there are some steps you can take now to help you get through it. Here are some suggestions.

Get active. Do some form of weight-bearing, aerobic exercise for 30 minutes at least three times a week, and more if possible. Weight-bearing activities—such as walking or running—help increase or maintain bone density. Aerobic exercise, the kind that gets your heart rate up continuously for at least 20 to 30 minutes, will also help keep your cholesterol level down and boost your feelings of well-being, Dr. Walsh says.

Eat less fat. Watch your fat intake: 25 percent or less of the calories you eat should come from fat, experts say. Eating a diet low in saturated fats will help bring your cholesterol level down.

Kick the butts. Smoking can worsen any menopausal symptoms you have, Dr. Walsh says. Smoking not only brings on menopause sooner, it also reduces the small amount of estrogen women do have after menopause. In addition to making you feel better at menopause, quitting the cigarette habit will also be better for your bone health—you'll have more estrogen available to maintain your bone strength.

Consume calcium. Get enough calcium to keep your bones strong and healthy. After age 35, women begin to lose about 1 percent of their bone mass per year. The Daily Value for calcium for premenopausal women is 1,000 milligrams, but some doctors recommend getting between 1,000 and 1,200 milligrams. An eight-ounce glass of 1 percent low-fat milk and one cup of low-fat yogurt with fruit contain about 300 milligrams each. Three ounces of canned sockeye salmon, with bones, contains about 203 milligrams, and a half-cup of tofu contains about 258 milligrams.

Calcium supplements are another option. When deciding how many supplements to take, read the label to see how much "elemental" or "bioavailable" calcium each tablet contains; that's the number of milligrams your body will actually absorb. Take the supplements with food and a glass of water to help your body absorb them easily and efficiently, says Kendra Kaye, M.D., clinical assistant professor of medicine at the University of Pennsylvania School of Medicine and attending physician at Graduate Hospital, both in Philadelphia.

Watch your cholesterol. Ask your doctor to check your cholesterol levels to make sure you are in the healthy range, says Dr. Walsh. She should measure the ratio of your total cholesterol to your good cholesterol, or HDL. A total cholesterol/HDL cholesterol ratio below 3.5 indicates that you are at low risk for a heart attack. A ratio between 3.5 and 6.9 means you are at moderate risk, and a ratio over 7.0 means you are at high risk. Menopause can cause your ratio to go up, because levels of LDL (bad cholesterol) go up and levels of HDL (good cholesterol) go down.

Monitor your symptoms. See your doctor if you have PMS and your symptoms are getting worse; you may have begun menopause, says Dr. Klutznick. Your doctor can perform a follicle-stimulating hormone test to determine whether that is the case.

Talk to Mom. If the uncertainty of menopause weighs on your mind, talk to your mother about it. It's not uncommon for women to follow the same pattern as their mothers, says Dr. Walsh, especially if they have a similar health history.

...And to your spouse. Share information you learn about menopause with your husband, says Dr. Klutznick. One way to do that is to ask him to read a book or two on menopause, she says. Some books have chapters just for men.

Savor the moment. Appreciating where you are in your life and enjoying it can make the menopausal transition easier, says Borton.

Taking Charge of the Change

Don't just sit back and worry, or try to ignore it. Here are tips to help you cope.

Reach out. "Talk to other women," says Dr. Klutznick. Find out what symptoms they're having, what causes them difficulty and what they do to cope. A lot of women are doing their own research and information-gathering, and they can be a tremendous resource for you, she says.

Find a mentor. Some older women who have been through menopause can serve as wonderful mentors, says Borton. Find a woman 10 to 15 years older who's living a lifestyle you admire and talk to her about what has meaning in her life. Make her a role model.

Know your options. Talk to your doctor about your symptoms and options for dealing with them. Deciding to take hormones is a very individual decision, experts say. Talk to several doctors if you need to, Dr. Klutznick says, until you find one you are comfortable with and who is willing to respect what you want to do to manage your menopause.

Stay connected. "Women need to have a community of other women," says Dr. Klutznick. This can help you feel connected and productive during this transitional time, she says. So join a book club or take art lessons or a course that stimulates your intellect, she says.

Expect sexual changes. Some women find that sex is not as passionate but becomes more affectionate. And this can be fine, since their mate's testosterone levels may be dropping as well, lowering his sex drive. Some women also find that certain places on the body that used to be highly sensitive are less so, and that other places that were not sensitive now are, says Dr. Klutznick.

Explore sexual options. Try to stay sexually active, doctors say. Not having sex can cause your vagina to change in size and elasticity, which can make sex painful. Communicate to your partner the changes you are feeling and explore new and different ways to have sex that may be more comfortable.

You may take longer to lubricate than you used to. Besides allowing yourself more time, you can also use water-based vaginal lubricants. Try K-Y Jelly or Replens, which are available in drugstores.

If you do not have a partner, masturbation helps promote circulation and moistness in the vagina, helping it to maintain its size and elasticity, says Dr. Klutznick.

Consider herbal remedies. Black cohosh, blue cohosh, sarsaparilla, wild yam root and dong quai are among some of the herbs doctors often recommend to alleviate menopausal symptoms. These herbs contain phytoestrogens, plant sources of estrogen similar to that produced in the body.

The levels of phytoestrogens found in these herbs are lower than the doses of estrogen in HRT and are believed by some doctors to relieve menopausal symptoms without causing harmful side effects. Consult with your doctor before using these remedies.

Do Women Doctors Take Estrogen?

Wondering whether hormone replacement therapy is right for you? Here's how some top female physicians made this sometimes-difficult choice.

Ask your doctor for advice about hormone therapy after menopause, and she may tell you something like this: "On the one hand, estrogen cures hot flashes and it probably reduces risk of osteoporosis and heart disease. On the other hand, estrogen taken without a progestogen—either the natural hormone progesterone or a synthetic form called a progestin—increases the risk of uterine cancer. And it's possible that either estrogen alone or estrogen and a progestogen together increase risk of breast cancer."

Does this sound confusing? You're not alone: Lots of women feel the same way. The fact is, making the right choice about whether to take hormone replacement therapy (HRT) is often tough. And it's all the tougher because the decision is so important. There's also no one-size-fits-all formula for making the right choice, because you have to consider personal factors that are unique to you as well as medical facts that apply to most women.

So how do women doctors—the most medically sophisticated women in the country—make their own personal decisions about hormone therapy after menopause? What circumstances influence their choices, and how do they weigh the risks and benefits of HRT?

The editors of *Prevention* magazine talked with dozens of women doctors across the country, all over age 45 and prominent in different medical specialties. To their surprise, the most important factor in deciding for or against HRT was usually not long-term lowering of risk for things like bone loss or heart disease or even the possibility of some increased risk. It was quality of life. The real question was "Will HRT improve my life right now?" (For information on weighing risk factors, see "What Women Doctors Tell Their Patients" on page 46.)

It's worth noting that most of the physicians interviewed who choose to take hormone therapy have had hysterectomies. This may not be representative of women in general.

Presented here are eight of the best interviews out of all those we conducted. Almost two-thirds of these postmenopausal women take HRT. (In the general population, however, approximately 15 to 25 percent of menopausal or postmenopausal women take HRT.)

Physicians Who Take HRT

SYDNEY BONNICK, M.D. *Director of Osteoporosis Services, Texas Woman's University, Denton; research professor at Texas Woman's University's Center for Research on Women's Health*

I went through a natural menopause when I was 38, which by anyone's standards is young. My ovaries simply stopped functioning. I was having hot flashes, menstrual irregularities, trouble concentrating and difficulty sleeping. Plus my memory was poor. My gynecologist told me it was stress and that I was too young for menopause. But to me, it was clear that something else was happening.

Finally we confirmed that it was menopause. Having heard, over the years, complaints of similar symptoms from menopausal patients, I felt confident that my symptoms were related to estrogen deficiency. I didn't hesitate to begin estrogen daily and progestin 12 days of the month. The progestin was necessary to prevent an increased risk of cancer of the uterus, which might develop if I were to take estrogen alone.

It was wonderful. The problems stopped, and my sense of well-being returned. But during the progestin days, I tended to feel not as well, which is not an unusual complaint. And I started having trouble with excessive bleeding and cramping. That turned out to be partly caused by fibroid tumors in my uterus, stimulated to grow by the estrogen.

After much time trying to control the bleeding, I finally threw in the towel and had a hysterectomy. No more fibroids or bleeding, and it eliminated the need for adding progestin to the estrogen therapy. I

WHAT WOMEN DOCTORS TELL THEIR PATIENTS

*A*n important factor in any decision about hormone replacement is quality of life, as several of the women doctors interviewed in this chapter point out.

But it's also important to look beyond present-day symptoms of menopause or hormone replacement and keep the long-term benefits and risks of estrogen in mind. All the physicians we interviewed—even those who chose not to use hormones themselves—emphasize that research suggests estrogen will probably turn out to be a lifesaver for tens of thousands of women at risk for heart disease and osteoporosis.

Marianne J. Legato, M.D., a cardiologist and associate professor of clinical medicine at Columbia University College of Physicians and Surgeons in New York City who does not take hormones herself, says she will prescribe them to women who have proven, strong risk factors for those diseases. "Of course," she says, "I give estrogen for intolerable symptoms of menopause, like hot flashes that make sleep difficult. But I will also sometimes prescribe it to prevent osteoporosis, if I have a patient with demonstrated thinning of the vertebra or hip bones. And I will prescribe it to a patient with a low HDL (good cholesterol below 40) plus two other risk factors for coronary artery disease, like hypertension and a parent who died of heart disease before age 55."

Other women physicians who are more positive about estrogen's benefits say they give it to women who don't have obvious risk factors for those diseases.

Valery T. Miller, M.D., professor of medicine and director of the

was happy as a clam. I can tell you absolutely that if I were to stop estrogen, I would have hot flashes, probably experience some bone loss and might be at increased risk for heart disease. I have stopped estrogen for brief periods, once because of an illness, and I know during that time that my quality of life was very poor. It does affect my intellect. I think that as medical science progresses, we will learn that both men's and women's intellectual functions, as well as emotions and sexuality, are affected by hormones.

I've often thought, what if I got breast cancer and my physician said I should not take estrogen? I think I would take it anyway be-

Lipid Research Clinic, George Washington University Medical Center, in Washington, D.C., argues, "No individual woman can know for sure whether she's going to develop osteoporosis or heart disease; even women without a family history can get those ailments. So it's a good idea for most women to take estrogen."

To identify your risk for osteoporosis and heart disease, talk to your physician. A bone density measurement at menopause is a good idea.

The sticky part is that you will also have to consider your risk for breast cancer. Currently scientists suspect that there's a small increased risk of breast cancer that is associated with long-term use of either estrogen alone or estrogen in combination with a progestogen. It's really an unanswered question; that's why most physicians we interviewed said they would warn a woman with a personal or strong family history of breast cancer to avoid hormones.

All the doctors we talked to agreed to one point: Each woman must be carefully and individually assessed. Wilma Bergfeld, M.D., a dermatologist and head of the Section of Dermatopathology and Dermatological Clinical Research at the Cleveland Clinic and associate clinical professor of dermatology at Case Western Reserve University School of Medicine in Cleveland, told us that if she has a patient considering estrogen and there are any special health concerns, she doesn't hesitate to consult other specialists. "I see it as my mission to talk to patients about safety precautions and inquire about hereditary and personal risk factors. With that, I can select patients who need reviews by gynecologists and breast centers before I'll give them hormones."

cause I know how profoundly my quality of life is affected without estrogen. Barring something strange, I will take it the rest of my life. There's nothing unnatural about a woman having estrogen in her system. I think we are very naive to assume estrogen's only role has to do with reproduction or sexual function. A woman of 50 today can expect to live an additional 30 years; asking her to live all that time in a hormone-deficient state is very strange. If your adrenal glands fail, we give you cortisone. If your thyroid gland fails, you need thyroid hormone replacement. So why do we view the failure of the ovaries differently?

VALERY T. MILLER, M.D. *Professor of medicine and director, Lipid Research Clinic, George Washington University Medical Center, Washington, D.C.*

I'm a clinical researcher in estrogen and progesterone use. I study it and write about it and am a big proponent of it. I didn't need it until I was 55. That's when my first and only symptom of menopause began: irregular heavy bleeding. Cancer was found in my uterus. So I had a hysterectomy and total oophorectomy (removal of the ovaries) at 55. Fortunately, the cancer was confined to a small area of the uterus.

At that time, just three years ago, it was considered a new and strange idea to allow women who had had cancer to take estrogen. I didn't go on it right away. It took two weeks for the hysterectomy and oophorectomy to affect me symptomatically. But two weeks after my surgery, I was suffering from sleeplessness, waking every hour on the hour at night. It was a very interesting experience, since I'd read about this in menopausal women for so long.

I called up my doctor and said, "I don't want to wait, let's get on with this; I'd like to have my estrogen." She said yes. I didn't need a progestogen—used to protect the lining of the uterus, or endometrium, from excessive tissue growth and cancer—since I didn't have a uterus.

I think I will always want estrogen, at least until research shows me there is a need to stop. I believe it improves the quality of my life by completely relieving symptoms I once had. I'm a large woman, so I probably won't have osteoporosis, and I don't have other risk factors for heart disease. But I think estrogen is a natural thing. I think women should have estrogen in their bodies until they die, just as men have testosterone. It's an oversight in nature to allow us to live the last 30 years of our lives without estrogen.

WILMA BERGFELD, M.D. *Dermatologist; head, Section of Dermatopathology and Dermatological Clinical Research, Cleveland Clinic; associate clinical professor of dermatology, Case Western Reserve University School of Medicine, Cleveland*

My specialty deals with hormone disorders in women. Estrogen therapy is important for many of these women. Treating women for the past 25 years, I've seen that estrogen is restorative to skin, hair and nails. Without estrogen, females cannot maintain the viability of their skin. Estrogen also maintains the health of vaginal mucosa, maintains pubic hair and, of course, reduces the risk of osteoporosis. Menopausal depression can also be reversed with estrogen. I have no doubt that estrogen is very good for females. When I came into my menopausal years, there was no hesitation in taking estrogen. A progestin was not needed because I'd had a hysterectomy.

The difficult question is, how much is enough? I still haven't found a dose I like. My endocrinologist tells me I need more to get all the benefits; my gynecologist tells me that for safety's sake, I need a lower dose. The more estrogen, the better skin, hair and nails. This is a dilemma for women and their physicians.

MARY K. BEARD, M.D. *Gynecologist; associate clinical professor of obstetrics and gynecology, University of Utah, Salt Lake City; author,* Menopause and the Years Ahead

My views in favor of estrogen came out of my special interest in older women. I was an internist for 16 years. I felt that older women were not being taken care of, and that was the reason I went back into training to become a gynecologist, about 14 years ago. I focused my research on estrogen replacement therapy, which, at that time, was not favored.

After reading all of the research that had been published around the world, I came to the conclusion that estrogen was very beneficial, not the bad drug people said it was.

I started estrogen when I became symptomatic, a year before I became fully menopausal. I was having hot flashes, especially at night, which interfered with my sleep. Also, I was feeling a little blue, and my thinking was not quite on target. I began with the smaller patch, which delivered a lower dose—all I needed for that year. As I hit full-blown menopause, it became apparent that that wasn't quite enough, so I raised the dose. I'd had a hysterectomy, so I didn't need a progestogen. I do have a risk for osteoporosis, and that just confirmed my decision. There's no cardiovascular disease in my family. Still, I feel estrogen is benefiting me, and I plan to take it for a lifetime, because I know the protective effects it has.

MARCELLE WILLOCK, M.D. *Anesthesiologist; professor and chair, Department of Anesthesiology, Boston University School of Medicine*

My periods were regular, and I hadn't reached menopause when I had a hysterectomy for bleeding fibroids about eight years ago, at age 48. I'd asked the surgeon to leave my ovaries; but he had to take one out. I didn't expect symptoms of menopause so quickly.

But they came on within about a month. You're sitting in a room and suddenly you're sweating, you're hot, you're trying to think about what you're doing, but you're distressed because it's so hot in the room. It was intolerable. After my first week of hot flashes, I said, "No way."

Estrogen worked like a charm, immediately. I've been taking it since then. Once, I forgot to take it on a long trip, and within a week the hot flashes started to come back. Boy, have I been compliant about taking my medication every day ever since.

I don't think much about the other benefits of estrogen therapy. I'm not at risk for osteoporosis, but there is a history of hypertension in my family. Women in my family have lived to their late seventies and eighties despite the hypertension; we all have to die of something, and I can't see myself worrying excessively about it. I take my antihypertensive medication and have my blood pressure checked regularly. I also have an annual pelvic exam and mammogram.

I plan to take estrogen at least until I retire. I'm not ready to deal with hot flashes while I'm still working, active and productive.

Physicians Who Don't Take HRT

MARIANNE J. LEGATO, M.D. *Cardiologist; associate professor of clinical medicine, Columbia University College of Physicians and Surgeons, New York City; author,* The Female Heart: The Truth about Women and Heart Disease

I tried estrogen and couldn't tolerate it. I had a reason to take it earlier than most women, namely a hysterectomy at 38 and by 42 I was beginning to have symptoms of menopause. I was put on hormone replacement, but it increased the frequency and intensity of my migraine headaches. I didn't take it very long!

When we decide that menopause is a disease and estrogen is the cure, I think there might be something flawed in that thinking. In fact, many studies show women's self-esteem and sense of well-being improve at menopause. When we look at who's depressed, mostly it's young women with small children, not postmenopausal women.

ELIZABETH A. PATTERSON, M.D. *Radiologist, Hospital of the University of Pennsylvania, Philadelphia, Department of Radiology; assistant professor of radiology, University of Pennsylvania School of Medicine; chair, Mammography Quality Assurance Advisory Committee, Food and Drug Administration*

I hardly noticed menopause. One day I woke up and observed that I wasn't going to the drugstore to buy tampons anymore! So I never took estrogen. I had no reason for it. I don't have any risk factors for osteoporosis—light-skinned women, especially with Scandinavian backgrounds, and Asian women are at the most risk for bone loss. I do have a family history of heart disease, but I'm not completely convinced yet that estrogen is the protective mechanism.

In the future, we may have some more answers. In the meantime, I will do all the good things that I can do. I watch the fat and cholesterol intake in my diet, and I walk regularly. I may be wrong, but it seems to me that individuals who are very active, exercise and watch their diet don't have as many problems with menopausal symptoms as women who just sit around. But the decision about estrogen must be an individual one.

MILLICENT HIGGINS, M.D. *Epidemiologist; deputy director of the Division of Epidemiology and Clinical Applications, National Heart, Lung and Blood Institute*

I don't take estrogen now, but I did in the past. I was about 59 and postmenopausal and was put on both estrogen and a progestin. I didn't really have any menopausal symptoms.

My gynecologist at that time was enthusiastic about women taking postmenopausal hormones—taking them until they're age 95, he said! He described menopause as an "estrogen-deficiency disease"!

I was on the therapy for three or four years. I didn't like the progestin's side effects, especially the bleeding following each cycle. I was on estrogen for about 21 days, then a progestin for about 5 days, which induced menstrual-like bleeding.

I wouldn't take estrogen alone (without a progestin) because of the increased risk of uterine cancer. I have not had a hysterectomy and am not at all keen on the idea of having regular endometrial biopsies. (*Note:* Women who take estrogen without natural progesterone or a progestin, but who have a uterus, need careful surveillance of the uterus. This includes an annual endometrial biopsy—removal of a sample of tissue from the lining of the uterus, which can be an uncomfortable office procedure.)

A few years ago, articles began appearing that cited a possible link between hormone therapy and breast cancer. What's more, my risk of heart disease is very low. I realized I was not likely to gain very much benefit from estrogen and might run some uncertain level of risk. I decided I was going to quit; that's what I did.

There are lots of other ways to reduce heart disease risk: not smoking, eating a low-fat diet with plenty of fruits and vegetables, exercising, drinking alcohol moderately, if at all. To protect my bones, I drink plenty of skim milk and I'm physically active. For me, that's the way to go. I don't take any medications for anything, and I've been extraordinarily healthy all my life. Perhaps it's because I was lucky enough to inherit some good genes. My mother recently celebrated her one-hundredth birthday; she's never taken hormone pills in her life.

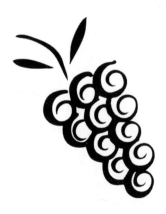

Do You Really Need a Hysterectomy?

There's a good chance you may not, say experts. Here's how to make the decision that's right for you.

*Y*ou know what a hysterectomy is. It's a surgical procedure in which a woman's uterus, and sometimes her ovaries, are removed. And you probably know that a lot of women have the operation and that the surgery has a reputation for being performed unnecessarily.

But you may not know what you would do if your doctor said, "You need a hysterectomy."

A Controversial "Cure"

Hysterectomies are the second most common operation performed in the United States, behind cesarean sections. From 1988 through 1991, an average of 564,000 hysterectomies a year were done. The surgery is performed most often on women in their early forties.

Controversy surrounds hysterectomy: Experts say about 25 percent of the operations are unnecessary. Gary Lipscomb, M.D., assistant professor in the Department of Gynecology at the University of Tennessee in Memphis, concedes that hysterectomies are sometimes performed when they're not medically warranted. In these cases, he says, doctors may err on the side of surgery instead of other approaches for a number of reasons.

"We are trained to be aggressive in managing disease," says Dr. Lipscomb. "And doing surgery is an active approach to problems, instead of a more passive approach. There's an old adage among surgeons in general that a chance to cut is a chance to cure."

Another reason some hysterectomies are done is that women suffering from heavy bleeding ask for the procedure as a way to stop it, says Dr. Lipscomb. Such hysterectomies may be medically unnecessary, but they may be appropriate as far as the woman is concerned, he says.

Also, some patients want treatment that will give them immediate results, so even when they are offered less invasive treatments that may take a while to be effective, they choose hysterectomy, he says.

Finally, some doctors may not offer alternative reproductive surgeries if they can't perform them as well, says Philip Brooks, M.D., clinical professor of obstetrics and gynecology at the University of California, Los Angeles, School of Medicine. "Not all doctors are competent in all procedures," he says. So if a doctor is better at removing the uterus than he is at removing fibroids, for example, he may offer hysterectomy alone.

The decision to have a hysterectomy is not an easy one. It's major surgery that involves incisions, a stay in the hospital, anesthesia and painful days afterward. It can also trigger physical, psychological and sexual changes, many of which doctors can't predict. If the ovaries are also removed, the surgery will cause a woman to have sudden, early menopause. And then there's the one definite consequence that's irreversible—the loss of the ability to bear children.

So women may wonder "Do I really need this procedure? Am I doing the right thing?" It's often hard to decide. And some women don't—they leave it up to their physician. "For some women who are having a lot of problems, they just want to get it over," says Linda Bernhard, R.N., Ph.D., associate professor of nursing and women's studies at Ohio State University in Columbus. "That puts women in a very vulnerable position to have some nice physician say, 'Well, we can fix you all up. We'll just take it all out, and then everything will be better.' "

But women can get involved, take control and make the decision that's right for them.

Not All Procedures Are Alike

Hysterectomy is most clearly warranted when a woman has cancer or serious, life-threatening complications during childbirth. Other conditions for which doctors might recommend or perform hysterectomies include fibroids, heavy bleeding, endometriosis, prolapsed uterus, pelvic pain and pelvic inflammatory disease, although when the surgery is necessary for these conditions is less clearly defined.

There are different types of hysterectomies. A total hysterectomy, for instance, removes the uterus and the cervix, while a partial hysterectomy removes only the uterus.

There are also different methods of doing a hysterectomy. In an abdominal hysterectomy, the uterus is removed through an incision in the abdomen. In a vaginal hysterectomy, the uterus is removed through an incision in the vagina. The vaginal surgery is less invasive, and recovery is easier than with the abdominal procedure.

In the 1990s, new techniques have been developed using laparoscopy. During the procedure, a laparoscope, a surgical microscope at the end of a viewing tube, is inserted through an incision in the navel, allowing physicians to view the woman's reproductive area, says Dr. Lipscomb. They can then determine whether a vaginal procedure would be likely to be effective.

In cases where a traditional vaginal hysterectomy might prove difficult to do, miniature operating instruments can be inserted through other small openings in the abdomen and the uterus removed vaginally under laparoscopic guidance. This is known as a laparoscopic-assisted hysterectomy.

In any of these procedures, doctors may recommend the removal of one or both ovaries in a procedure called an oophorectomy. Some doctors advocate removing the ovaries in women who have finished bearing children in order to prevent ovarian cancer. Other medical professionals recommend leaving the ovaries in as long as possible because they supply estrogen, which plays a role in preventing osteoporosis and heart disease, as well as androgen, which influences a woman's sex drive.

About the Alternatives

The thing to remember about hysterectomy is that a lot of times it's not the only possible treatment, says Paula Bernstein, M.D., Ph.D., attending physician at Cedars-Sinai Medical Center in Los Angeles. There are usually other treatment alternatives for fibroids, heavy bleeding, pelvic pain, endometriosis, prolapsed uterus and pelvic inflammatory disease.

Fibroids are the reason for about 30 percent of hysterectomies.

Alternatives include leaving fibroids alone or removing them through myomectomy, which leaves the uterus in place.

Heavy bleeding, the problem that leads to 20 percent of hysterectomies, can often be treated with medication or a procedure called endometrial ablation, in which the lining of the uterus is removed but the organ is left intact. Endometriosis can be treated with drugs as well, or the diseased tissue alone can be removed using laparoscopy.

Fifteen percent of hysterectomies are performed for prolapsed uterus, in which the uterus literally starts to fall. Women who develop a prolapsed uterus can ask their doctors about exercises called Kegels, which help to strengthen the uterine muscle. (See also "How to Kegel Correctly" on page 79.) They can also ask about a pessary, a device that is inserted in the vagina—much like a diaphragm—to hold the uterus in place.

Obstetrical complications, such as hemorrhaging during childbirth and gynecologic cancer, are the reasons for about 11 percent of hysterectomies. For these conditions, there's usually no alternative. "Those are the life-threatening reasons," says Susan Haas, M.D., assistant professor of obstetrics and gynecology at Harvard Medical School.

In other cases, though, whether a woman has a hysterectomy is ultimately up to her. "In my opinion, since the woman lives with all the risks and all the benefits, she's the one who makes the decision," says Dr. Haas. "We should term this 'elective hysterectomy.' That reinforces the concept that it's an option or a choice and that the final decision-making power lies with the woman. It also implies that she can make that decision at any point," she says.

Even in the case of cancer, if a woman feels she's not quite ready for the surgery, it probably can wait a day or two, says Marvel Williamson, R.N., Ph.D., professor of nursing and director of the School of Nursing at Park College in Parkville, Missouri. Meanwhile, women need to take the time to find out their options, adds Dr. Bernhard.

Other Important Considerations

Hysterectomy may cause a woman to have an early menopause even if she does not have her ovaries removed. If you're a candidate for surgery and you're still in your childbearing years, consider the fact that you will no longer be able to have children. Hot flashes and vaginal dryness, two other side effects of menopause, may also occur.

Women who undergo hysterectomy can also experience urinary tract symptoms such as frequent urination and urinary incontinence, as well as deepening of the voice and weight gain. These physical changes are the result of declining estrogen levels.

Some studies indicate that women feel depressed after a hysterectomy, but whether the operation itself causes depression is unclear. "Our society still has this negative perception that hysterectomy is going to make you something less. If women internalize that, then they may feel depressed," says Dr. Bernhard.

Other studies show that depression after a hysterectomy may be no more typical than depression about bodily changes that can occur after other types of surgery. And some studies reveal that women are less depressed after hysterectomy than they were before, when they suffered with problems such as heavy bleeding and pain.

Some women say they've experienced positive physical changes, reporting restored vigor because they're no longer bleeding heavily and suffering pain. The operation can often end anemia as well. "I've heard women say they just feel so much better. The physical improvement in their health is often the greatest reward," says Dr. Bernhard.

While studies indicate that women have these positive responses in the short term, more study is needed on the long-term effects, says Dr. Bernhard.

Women may experience sexual changes after hysterectomy because they feel different about their bodies and have anxiety about resuming sex. For some women, the orgasm experience changes. "It's not that they don't have orgasms, they just are different," says Dr. Bernhard.

Women may also have a lower sex drive, particularly if they've had their ovaries removed, says Dr. Williamson.

The Best Advice: Take an Active Role

If you are a candidate for hysterectomy, weigh your decision carefully. Here's some help.

Find the right doctor. Look for a doctor you can talk to, who understands what you're going through, answers your questions and will do what you want, says Nancy Petersen, R.N., director of the Endometriosis Treatment Center at St. Charles Medical Center in Bend, Oregon. If your doctor tells you that you need a hysterectomy but it doesn't seem right to you, see another doctor. Hysterectomy is often overkill for endometriosis, she says.

Explore the alternatives. There are usually other options to hysterectomy, experts say. Ask your doctor what they are, says Dr. Williamson.

Get a second—and third—opinion. "Don't let any one physician tell you this is what you should do," says Dr. Bernhard.

Ask lots of questions. Ask your doctor which particular procedure will be done and why, says Dr. Brooks. Find out how much experience your doctor has with the procedure she is suggesting.

Decide what's important. Set your priorities, says Dr. Bernstein. Ask yourself "How debilitating is the pain? How much is it interfering with my lifestyle? Do I want to have children? Would I feel comfortable about adopting?"

Think your decision through. Take time to make your decision, says Dr. Bernhard. "There's probably no rush," she says.

After the Surgery

If you decide to have a hysterectomy, ask your doctor whether the less invasive vaginal surgery is right for you. "If there is a choice, a vaginal is always the safer, more comfortable way to go," says Dr. Williamson.

Find out whether your doctor has experience using the laparoscope, since its use in hysterectomy is fairly new. Keep in mind, though, that if you have ovarian cancer, an abdominal hysterectomy is usually the only option, says Dr. Lipscomb.

Here are some things you can do to make the surgery easier.

Involve your mate. Studies show that men often view their partners differently after hysterectomy, so "we need to help him understand," says Dr. Williamson. "Don't be afraid to ask him 'What fears do you have about my hysterectomy? How do you think my surgery will affect our sex life?' " You may have to take the initiative in getting

EIGHT MUST-ASK QUESTIONS

Deciding whether or not to have a hysterectomy is difficult. Explore all your options by asking questions of your doctor. Here are some to begin with.

- Why are you recommending a hysterectomy?
- Is there an option other than hysterectomy?
- What are the pros and cons of a hysterectomy for my problem?
- Do you recommend removal of my ovaries? If so, why? What are the risks and benefits of keeping them? The risks and benefits of removing them?
- Why are you recommending an abdominal (or vaginal) hysterectomy?
- Are you planning to use a laparoscope? If so, how much of the surgery will you do with the laparoscope?
- How many procedures like mine have you done with a laparoscope?
- When you do the procedure, will there be another surgeon present who is experienced in using a laparoscope for hysterectomy?

the conversation going. Sometimes having the partner sit in on doctor's visits can help.

Get support. Talk to your female friends or join a support group. "Sometimes women find talking about it with other women helps more than talking with just their partner," says Dr. Williamson. Ask your doctor or call a local hospital for support groups near you.

Grieve your loss. "As for any loss, the grief process needs to be expressed," says Dr. Williamson. "If women can't talk about it or cry about it, the feelings of grief will come out in some other way. Give yourself permission to talk about it." Find someone, say a friend or therapist, who will go through it with you, she says.

First, be intimate alone. After surgery, women should "have their first orgasm alone," says Dr. Williamson. They should masturbate the first time so they can get used to any new sensations, she says. "It lets them know that everything still works and that it doesn't hurt to get turned on and have an orgasm." It also lets them do it without their partner pressuring them or without feeling like they have to perform, she says.

Make sex new. When women who've had a hysterectomy are ready to start intercourse again, the couple needs to pretend it's their very first time having sex, says Dr. Williamson. "They need to allow her to be in control, to have as long a foreplay session as possible," she says. Many women are concerned that sex will be painful, so taking it slow can help, she says. And don't be afraid to use artificial lubricating jellies, she says. Products to consider for vaginal dryness include K-Y Jelly and Replens (available in pharmacies).

Use sex to heal. Try to have sex as soon as you can after the surgery, says Dr. Williamson. She recommends that women wait 10 to 14 days for the incision to heal. Part of the healing process after surgery is the development of scar tissue, and if women wait too long, the scar tissue in the pelvic cavity and around the vaginal incision can become very tough, making sex more uncomfortable, she says. Having sex can minimize the scar tissue toughness, because the area gets increased circulation and expands during engorgement.

"We would like women to resume gentle intercourse between the two- and four-week period, if possible," she says. Women should try to have sex at least twice a week until the healing process is complete, she says, which can take as long as three months. "I just don't recommend that women who have had regular intercourse in their lives let that go," she says.

Expand your sexual repertoire. Before the surgery, get in the habit of varying your sexual techniques, because you probably will have to do so after the surgery, at least at first, says Dr. Williamson. "If it feels like it's part of your sex life to try new positions and new settings, it won't be as much of a shock when you do it after the surgery," she says.

Try Kegels. Many women say the pleasurable feeling of needing to be filled that they experienced during sex is no longer there after hysterectomy, says Dr. Williamson. Performing Kegels during sex can help women achieve that feeling, she says, because they help lengthen and lift the vagina.

Normally, Kegels can be done anywhere; you simply tighten your pelvic floor muscles as if you are trying to keep from urinating, hold for up to ten seconds, then release. After hysterectomy, do Kegels during sex. Besides strengthening the vaginal muscles, Kegels will enhance the feeling of pressure on the penis, Dr. Williamson says.

Outwitting Ovarian Cancer

Doctors say there are new ways you can help reduce your risk of developing this killer, even if it runs in your family.

*U*ntil recently, the news on ovarian cancer has been pretty scary. Although the disease is fairly uncommon—striking one woman in 70, compared with one in 9 for breast cancer—fewer than half survive. But now a different kind of news is breaking. A revolution has occurred in understanding the genetics of the disease, treatments are improving and doctors are beginning to get a clearer picture of its causes.

While ovarian cancer most often occurs in women over 60, researchers have found that where there is a strong family history of ovarian cancer, daughters are developing the disease approximately a decade earlier than their mothers did, possibly because they've been exposed to more pollution or other environmental risks, says M. Steven Piver, M.D., head of the Department of Gynecologic Oncology at Roswell Park Cancer Institute in Buffalo.

Most important, whether or not you have a family history, doctors are learning, it's during your twenties, thirties and forties that you can do the most to offset your risk. Here are some questions you may have—and the answers doctors want you to have.

Q. *My mother had ovarian cancer. Does that mean I'm destined to have it, too?*

A. No. Although family history puts you most at risk, it's important to consider *how many* family members have been affected. If one close relative (mother, sister, aunt, grandmother) has had the disease, your chance of developing it is about 5 to 7 percent—only moderately higher than the 1.4 percent for a woman with no family history. But if two or three close relatives have had ovarian cancer, your family may be part of a hereditary cancer syndrome. Although this is rare, the risk of ovarian cancer for women in this category may be as high as 40 to 50 percent.

Keep in mind, though, that it may be hard to know your family history. The disease was not always spoken about so openly. Frequently, women referred to problems "down there," which could have meant ovarian cancer or something else.

Q. *What if the disease runs on my father's side?*

A. That counts just as much, according to Henry T. Lynch, M.D., chairman of the Department of Preventive Medicine at Creighton University in Omaha, Nebraska.

Q. *Researchers recently announced that they'd found the gene implicated in ovarian cancer. Does this mean doctors can now tell if you've inherited it?*

A. Yes—and no. They've found the exact location of a gene called BRCAI, which is implicated in some ovarian cancer and some kinds of breast cancer, but for now the test is used only for research. It will be several years before you can walk into your doctor's office and have a simple blood test to tell whether you have the gene.

Q. *Besides family history, what else puts women at higher risk?*

A. Those who've never had children or who've had only one child are 50 percent more likely to develop the disease. Conversely, having two or three children appears to lower your chances substantially. The probable reason: Pregnancy interrupts the constant flow of eggs and gives the ovaries a chance to rest. Over time, as eggs continue to erupt out of the ovaries, the ovarian surface lining breaks and must repair itself. This excessive lifetime cyclical change paves the way for a cancer mutation. Researchers have also noted that women of northern European heritage are 40 percent more likely to get ovarian cancer than African Americans, Hispanics or Native Americans.

ONE WOMAN'S TRIUMPH OVER OVARIAN CANCER

*L*ong before Gilda Radner focused national attention on ovarian cancer, Dianne Schuh, an elementary school teacher in her early forties from Orchard Park, New York, was intimately familiar with the disease. In 1966 Schuh's mother was diagnosed with it and died a short time later. "I was only fifteen at the time, but I realized then that if it could happen to my mother it could happen to me, too," she says.

By 1985 five more women—two aunts and three cousins, all on Schuh's mother's side—had died from ovarian cancer, most of them in their forties. "Science hadn't found the genetic link yet, but we knew every woman in my family was at risk," says Schuh.

Just before Schuh's aunt died, she urged her niece to have her ovaries removed. Schuh decided to do it. "It made sense to me that if I didn't have ovaries, I couldn't get ovarian cancer," she says.

And so in 1985, at the age of 34, Schuh had a complete hysterectomy (today many women have only their ovaries removed). As a result of the operation, Schuh, who already had two daughters, went into menopause and was placed on estrogen replacement therapy to offset the symptoms. She was concerned about sex but knew the hormones would help. "I had tremendous support from my husband, and I'm happy to say things really haven't changed," she says. Most of all, she felt relieved. "I can't explain the burden that was lifted," she says. "My anxiety was completely gone."

Schuh, whose risk of developing ovarian cancer has dropped from 50 percent to 2 percent, has no regrets about the surgery, although because of her family history she's still monitored. She participates in genetic research and volunteers as a counselor on a cancer help line. "I hope that my efforts make my relatives' deaths more meaningful—that these women died for a reason," she says.

Q. *Recent studies have linked fertility drugs to ovarian cancer. Should women who took these drugs be alarmed?*

A. "I think they should take the reports seriously," says Noel Weiss, M.D., an epidemiologist at the University of Washington School of Public Health in Seattle and an author of one of the recent studies. "But we really need more data."

What researchers did find in the University of Washington study was that women who took the fertility drug clomiphene (Clomid,

Serophene) for a year or longer were 11 times more likely to contract ovarian cancer than nonusers. This would fit, say experts, since fertility drugs push the ovaries to turn out more eggs, irritating the ovarian lining and potentially increasing chances of a malignancy.

But cause and effect have not been absolutely established, researchers point out. It may be infertility itself that accounts for the higher incidence of ovarian cancer in fertility-drug patients.

Q. *What if I'm contemplating taking fertility drugs?*

A. It seems safe to use them for no more than six cycles, advises Leon Speroff, M.D., professor of obstetrics and gynecology at Oregon Health Sciences University in Portland. Women in the University of Washington study who took clomiphene for less than 12 months were at no increased risk. Nor is there much benefit to taking them longer—the chances of conceiving after 4 to 6 months on ovulation-stimulating drugs such as Clomid are slim.

Q. *Any other risks women should pay attention to?*

A. Diet. Just as with breast and colon cancer, saturated fats (especially whole milk and red meat) may contribute to ovarian cancer.

The ovaries may also be affected by substances that make their way into the body through the vagina—such as talcum powder, which, chemically, is related to asbestos. "Studies have shown talc granules in ovarian tumors, suggesting more research needs to be done," says Carolyn D. Runowicz, M.D., director of gynecologic oncology at Albert Einstein College of Medicine and Montefiore Medical Center in New York. Powders made with cornstarch appear to be safe.

Q. *I have a family history of ovarian cancer. Is there anything I can do to lower my risk?*

A. Take the Pill. Oral contraceptives, which halt the release of eggs, can cut your risk by as much as 50 percent if taken for five years; after ten years, your risk may be lower than that of a woman with no family history of ovarian cancer who hasn't taken the Pill.

Q. *Anything besides taking the Pill?*

A. Tying off the fallopian tubes (sterilization surgery) also seems to lessen your risk, according to a recent Harvard study. Researchers suspect this may work because the ovaries are sealed off and therefore protected from foreign substances and environmental contaminants.

A more controversial measure (and one reserved for highest-risk women) is prophylactic oophorectomy, in which the ovaries are removed as a preventive measure.

Q. *Why is ovarian cancer so difficult to detect early?*

A. The symptoms—bloating, heartburn, pelvic pain, cramping, fatigue—are vague: They could also be from indigestion or a bad case of PMS. With advanced ovarian cancer, though, the abdominal swelling is pronounced and gets progressively worse, you have a decrease in appetite and you lose weight. PMS is more likely to cause bloating that comes and goes, food cravings and temporary weight gain. Nonetheless, says Vicki L. Seltzer, M.D., chairman of obstetrics and gynecology at Long Island Jewish Medical Center in New Hyde Park, New York, if you have any of these symptoms for more than three to four weeks, you should see a doctor.

Q. *Can doctors detect ovarian cancer during a regular pelvic exam?*

A. They may be able to tell if your ovaries feel enlarged (that's why it's important for all women to have annual exams), but it takes surgery and a biopsy to confirm a malignancy. If your gynecologist suspects an abnormality, you'll probably have a transvaginal sonogram, in which a probe is inserted into the vagina to get a closer look at the ovaries and search for tumors.

Q. *Are ultrasound exams recommended as a screening?*

A. Only for women with at least one first-degree (mother, sister, daughter) or two second-degree (aunt, grandmother) relatives who've had the disease. Too many of the masses picked up in these tests prove to be benign, according to studies. Jack van Nagell, M.D., director of gynecologic oncology at the University of Kentucky in Lexington, has conducted ultrasound tests on some 7,000 women, and although he calls the technology "very promising," he feels more data is needed.

Q. *Why did the National Institutes of Health come out against using the blood test CA-125 for routine screening?*

A. Unfortunately, the test—which measures a protein shed by ovarian tumors—isn't reliable enough to warrant mass screening along the lines of a Pap smear for cervical cancer or a mammogram for breast cancer, says Dr. Seltzer, who was chairman of the panel.

Although a high CA-125 might indicate ovarian cancer and *is* an accurate gauge for recurrences in women who've already been diagnosed, you might have a high CA-125 for any number of other reasons. These include endometriosis (growth of uterine tissue outside the uterus), pelvic inflammatory disease, fibroids, cysts, even menstruation. "Women went to their doctors in droves demanding CA-125 tests after Gilda Radner died," says Dr. Seltzer. "As a result of false positives, lots of women had surgery they would have been better off without."

Q. *If my blood test is normal, does that mean I'm okay?*

A. False negatives are an even bigger problem. The test *misses* 50 percent of early-stage ovarian tumors and, more worrisome, 20 percent of tumors in advanced stages. Researchers are working on a more accurate test, however.

Q. *If ovarian cancer is diagnosed, then what?*

A. A woman will usually undergo surgery to remove her ovaries as well as her uterus and fallopian tubes. Then she's treated with chemotherapy. When the cancer is confined to the ovaries (stage I), nearly 90 percent of patients survive. Survival is 70 percent when the cancer has spread into the uterus and fallopian tubes (stage II), but in stage III, when it has spread to the abdomen, survival drops to 15 percent. However, doctors are optimistic that new chemotherapy drugs may improve these statistics. Since the anti-cancer drug Taxol has been used for advanced cases of ovarian cancer, patient survival has increased by about 9 to 12 months.

For More Information

If two or more close relatives have had ovarian cancer, it's a good idea to be in the care of a gynecologic oncologist. For a list of qualified specialists in your area, call the Gynecologic Cancer Foundation information hotline at 1-800-444-4441.

To better understand the genetics of the disease, researchers at the Roswell Park Cancer Institute in Buffalo are keeping a registry of families at high risk. To add your family—or to speak with volunteers who have faced ovarian cancer—call 1-800-OVARIAN.

Breast Protection at Your Fingertips

Examining your breasts can save your life, yet many of us aren't sure how. The key: practice, practice, practice.

*B*reast self-examination (BSE) is among our most powerful tools against breast cancer. The combination of monthly BSE, annual physical exams and regular mammograms forms a "screen" through which few early cancers can pass undetected. And a recent study suggests that, with adequate BSE training, women can do a more thorough exam than most doctors.

That's the good news. The bad news is that the American Cancer Society (ACS) estimates that a mere 18 to 36 percent of all women do BSE. "Why?" we asked. Here's what women told us—and what the nation's top breast cancer experts say you should know.

I'm afraid of what I might find. "I think every woman is afraid of doing BSE—even me, and breast cancer is my specialty," says Janet Osuch, M.D., breast cancer surgeon and associate professor of surgery at Michigan State University in East Lansing. But, she adds, the odds are in women's favor. Fully 80 percent of all breast lumps aren't cancer—they're more likely to be harmless fluid-filled cysts, fibroadenomas or benign noncancerous tumors referred to as fibrocystic lumps.

The advantage of BSE is that a woman who does it regularly and thoroughly can detect lumps as small as one-quarter inch to one-half inch. If the lump is cancer, then there's a good chance she caught it early and can be effectively treated without losing her breast. The size of the tumor is the primary factor in evaluating women for lumpectomy—the breast-conserving surgical procedure in which the lump, the surrounding tissue and the lymph nodes under the arm are removed. "A woman who finds a one-quarter to one-half-inch lump has a 90 to 95 percent chance of having a lumpectomy instead of a mastectomy," says Jeanne Petrek, M.D., a breast surgeon at Memorial Sloan-Kettering Cancer Center in New York.

I have a mammogram every year. Mammograms are excellent screening tools (they can pick up tumors too small to be felt), but it's important to remember that they're not perfect, says Barnett Kramer, M.D., M.P.H., associate director of the early detection and community oncology program at the National Cancer Institute in Bethesda, Maryland. They do miss malignant tumors and miss a larger proportion in younger women.

"There's a small percentage of cancers that you might not actually see on a mammogram but that you can feel," explains Patti Wilcox, R.N., a nurse practitioner at the Breast Clinic at Johns Hopkins Oncology Center in Baltimore. This happens especially in younger women, whose breast tissue is dense with ducts and milk-producing glands that may be indistinguishable from tumors on mammogram film. Plus, there's a chance you could develop a tumor in the interval between mammograms.

That's why physical exams (and monthly breast self-exams, in particular) are so important. By palpating your breasts, your doctor may discover a lump the mammogram missed. And if you're trained in BSE and practice the method regularly, you've got yourself well-protected between office visits.

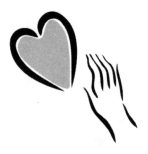

REMEMBERING NOT TO FORGET

*T*reat breast self-examination (BSE) like a standing appoint-ment—mark it on your calendar. If your periods come like clockwork, simply mark "BSE" in the square a week after the day your period's scheduled to begin each month. That's the time of the menstrual cycle when your breasts should be less painful and lumpy.

If your period's more unpredictable, or if you're postmenopausal, you may find it helpful to schedule your BSE session on the first of every month. Or tie it in with another monthly activity, like a stand-ing haircut appointment.

Research suggests that having a "BSE buddy" may help, too. That means pairing up with a close friend and agreeing to remind each other with a phone call or a note when it's time for your monthly exam.

I'm in my thirties. In fact, ACS suggests that women begin prac-ticing BSE at age 20. "While the risk of developing breast cancer at that age is very low, the earlier you get into the habit of doing self-exams, and the longer you do them, the more likely you will be able to discover a change in your breast early," says Terry Ades, R.N., director of nursing programs at ACS.

Another good reason to begin BSE early: Breast cancer doesn't strike just older women. "It's true that 75 percent of all cases are dis-covered in women age 50 and older. But about 46,000 women under 50 are diagnosed with breast cancer each year," Ades says. That's equal to all of the cases of invasive cervical cancer and uterine cancer combined.

"Women in their thirties are good about getting Pap smears regu-larly because they recognize they're at risk for cervical cancer—but the fact is, breast cancer in that age group is ten times more common than cervical cancer," Dr. Osuch notes.

It's hard to distinguish an abnormal lump in my generally lumpy breasts. "Your only responsibility is to look for a change in what you usually feel when you do your exam," says breast cancer specialist Wilcox. A nurse practitioner who trains women in BSE, Wilcox likens normal breast tissue to lumpy oatmeal. "What you're looking for is something that isn't consistent with the usual lumpy-oatmeal consistency of your breast tissue, whether it feels like a grape, a peanut or a piece of gravel," she says.

If you think you feel a new lump, but you're not certain, check the same area of your other breast for comparison. "Your other breast is your built-in point of reference," Dr. Osuch explains. "If you feel the same thing in the mirror-image location in the opposite breast, then what you're feeling is normal for you. That can be extraordinarily reassuring."

If the lump is in one breast only and it appears just before or during your period, repeat your self-exam seven days after the day your period began. Hormonal changes during the menstrual cycle naturally make breasts more lumpy—that's why experts recommend that premenopausal women do BSE a week postperiod, when breast tissue is back to normal. Don't be afraid to call your doctor if you have any doubt.

I've tried BSE, but I'm still not sure I know what I'm doing. Pamphlets, shower cards, even videos illustrating the basics of BSE can help remind us what to do. But most experts agree that the best way to learn BSE is during a one-on-one session with a qualified instructor.

Studies show that learning BSE in individual sessions practicing on silicone breast models is more effective in improving a woman's ability to detect breast lumps than learning through pamphlets or videos alone.

Generally, the jellylike silicone breast models are constructed to simulate healthy breast tissue, with abnormal lumps embedded in different sections (hidden under flesh-colored plastic, so you can't see them). Some of the lumps are pebble-hard; some soft, like a kitchen sponge. They can be fixed just under the skin, anchored deep, close to the rib cage, or they can move freely.

"Experiencing the feel of the different types of lumps can give you a better idea of what to look for," says Barbara Rimer, Dr.Ph., director of cancer prevention, detection and control research at Duke Comprehensive Cancer Center in Durham, North Carolina.

You should be aware, too, that there are different BSE palpation

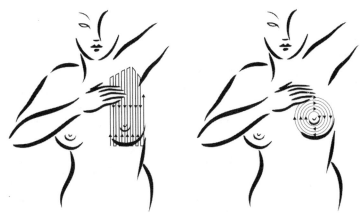

Best for breasts: The vertical-strip technique (left) involves an up-and-down motion with fingers rather than the traditional circular pattern (right). Including the entire breast area ups the odds of finding any suspicious lump.

patterns, including the traditional circular-pattern technique and the newer vertical-strip technique.

Research comparing the different BSE patterns shows that the vertical-strip technique is more effective. Women taught a method called MammaCare, which uses the vertical-strip technique, spend more time examining their breasts, cover more of the breast area and are able to detect more breast lumps (with fewer false alarms) than women who did BSE the traditional way. Not only that, women who were well-trained in the MammaCare method were able to pick out significantly more breast lumps in silicone models than a group of physicians and nurse practitioners. "You know your body better than anyone else," says Dr. Petrek. "If you put consistent effort into it, you could become a better breast examiner of your own breasts than I, or any other doctor, could be."

Here's how the vertical-strip technique works: Begin just under your collarbone, near your shoulder. Using your opposite hand, press with the pads of your fingers (not your fingertips) in a strip, along the outside of your breast. Work your way down to your bra line. Then slide over about a half-inch, and work your way back up to your collarbone. (The rows should overlap a bit, like they do when you're mowing a lawn.) Repeat the pattern until you hit the breastbone.

ONE WOMAN'S LIFESAVING LESSON

The author of this chapter recalls her lesson in breast self-examination. This is what she learned.

I confess: I had never performed a breast self-exam (BSE) before I got this assignment. Sure, I'd seen the pamphlets, and, perhaps inspired, pawed myself a couple of times in the shower. But I didn't feel much of anything (except maybe a little foolish), so I gave up.

But I'm not one to preach what I don't practice. So early on in my research, I went for a BSE training session with Carol Pilgrim, Ph.D., professor of psychology at the University of North Carolina at Wilmington. As a doctoral student in the early 1980s, Dr. Pilgrim helped develop a BSE method called MammaCare—which many breast experts say is the best lump detection system around.

Dr. Pilgrim led me to an examination room and left me to shed my shirt and lie back on the table with a soft paper sheet covering my torso. When she came back, she brought with her a breast model—a clear silicone breast rising out of a flat, square, equally squishy base. I could see the different textures of the pseudobreast tissue; some portions were completely smooth, others were wavy under the surface. There were also four lumps of different sizes at different depths. Dr. Pilgrim described the three parts of the MammaCare method, explaining that each should be practiced first on the model and then immediately on my own breast tissue to get an idea of how the method should feel.

With the three fingers of my right hand together (excluding the thumb and pinkie), in the Girl Scout salute formation, I learned the first part of the "palpation" technique: Press the skin, moving your hand in tiny circles "as if you're tracing the edges of a dime with your middle finger," Dr. Pilgrim explained. I tried it out on the model, immediately sensing a tiny lump lodged just under the skin. It felt just like a dried-up pencil eraser, too hard to do the job anymore.

The second part of the palpation was to apply different degrees of pressure. On the same patch of silicone skin, I made three circles: one lightly, on the surface, next at a midpoint in the breast, and the third

Then switch to the other breast. *Note:* The vertical-strip technique should be performed while lying on a bed. A small pillow or folded towel may be placed under the shoulder on the side of the breast being examined to center and flatten it.

pressing all the way down to the base. (Ouch! I thought.) Why use different pressures? Dr. Pilgrim showed me on the model how, when a lump is located at a midpoint in your breast, it can scoot right out from under your fingers if you press too hard—or if you press too lightly, you can miss a lump located deep in your breast, near your rib cage.

Now came the test: Another breast model, with a skin-colored, opaque coating, was produced. I was to examine it in its entirety, using the "vertical-strip technique" (see the text for an explanation), pointing out any lumps I would discover—with Dr. Pilgrim carefully watching my every move.

I found that I had to concentrate the entire time, and be extremely patient; when I started to hurry, my form fell apart. The verdict? My technique was okay, but I definitely needed practice. I got an A-plus in palpation pressure. But several times when I went to slide my hand into position for another palpation, I went a little too far—which means I would have missed an area if Dr. Pilgrim hadn't been there to correct me.

She also caught me a couple of times using the tips of my fingers—a common mistake—not the pads, she said. Keeping your fingers flat as you palpate allows you to cover more area. And I did miss one lump, one about the size of a pea, hiding directly under the nipple at the model's deepest part.

Then it was time for me to do a complete examination of my own breasts—both of them. I admit that during the entire session I was a bit embarrassed about palpating my bare breasts in front of a woman I'd just met half an hour ago. But Dr. Pilgrim was very understanding and put me at ease. I was struck by how different from the model my breasts feel; they don't quite spring back into place when I press into them, and their texture is much smoother. And I was happy to discover that the toughest pressure didn't hurt. During that training session and as I practiced later at home, however, I realized that I tend not to examine the area up by my collarbone as thoroughly as I should. I need to get used to the idea that my breast covers a large area across my chest.

This is different from the concentric-circle pattern you may have seen in some pamphlets. The circular method tends to leave out a large part of the breast—often the fleshy, upper-outer portion of the breast near your armpit, where tumors are typically found in large numbers.

"Your breast is much more than just the part that fits into a bra cup," Wilcox says. "It goes from your armpit to your breastbone, and from your collarbone to your bra line underneath your breast."

My breasts are large and difficult to examine. Larger breasts tend to fall to the outside when you're lying down, so they become thicker in that area and are more difficult to examine in depth. But, according to nurse practitioner Wilcox, there's a special position, which patients call the Scarlett O'Hara, that can help. To examine your left breast, lie on a bed on your right side, your left hip pointed up to the ceiling. Twist your upper torso and lean your left shoulder back on the bed. Place the back of your left hand on your forehead to flatten the outside of the breast, so you can examine it more easily. Examine the outer half of the breast from the armpit inward. When you've reached the nipple, lie flat on your back and continue to examine yourself from the nipple to the breast bone. Then repeat this process on the other breast.

It doesn't take a medical degree to do a good breast self-exam, adds Amy Langer, executive director of the National Alliance of Breast Cancer Organizations. Dr. Osuch agrees: "The fact remains, women who know their bodies well can, with their doctors, help fight breast cancer."

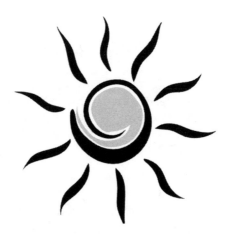

Understanding Urinary Incontinence

If coughing, sneezing or working out makes you spring a leak, you're not alone. So don't get embarrassed, get help.

*M*ary Pieratt first felt the embarrassing sensation of leaking urine, the clammy, soiled feeling of wet underwear, when she was eight years old, bouncing on the family trampoline. She never mentioned it to her sister or her mother. When it came time to play on the trampoline again, Pieratt secretly helped herself to her mother's menstrual supplies and padded her underwear. From then on, through her teens and twenties, she was incontinent every time she coughed, sneezed or went on a long run.

Though most of us associate urinary incontinence with old folks in nursing homes, the problem is much more common. By even the most conservative estimates, one in every ten women under the age of 65 is incontinent from time to time. Women in their twenties and thirties are nearly as vulnerable to the condition as those in their forties and fifties.

Women have been embarrassed to discuss this hidden problem. But that's changing. A decade ago, 11 out of 12 incontinent women never reported the problem to their doctors; now, about half do. "I can see the transition in my practice," says Nicolette Horbach, M.D., a urogynecologist at George Washington University Medical Center in Washington, D.C. "Young women come in after having the problem for only four to six months. They don't want to tolerate even a small amount of leakage."

Estimates of women's incontinence vary widely because physicians measure the problem not by the amount of urine that escapes but by how much it bothers the individual. For some women, even half a teaspoonful of urine is too much, especially if it happens two or three times a day. Others may tolerate leaks measuring half a cup, if they occur only once or twice a year.

What Causes Incontinence

There are several different kinds of incontinence, but the one that most often affects young women is known as stress incontinence. It's usually linked to weakness in the pelvic floor muscles and ligaments, which form a hammock of support for the bladder and the urethra (the tube through which the bladder empties), as well as the vagina and lower colon. Pregnancy contributes to incontinence, with high levels of the hormone progesterone relaxing muscles and ligaments. But pregnancy-related incontinence usually disappears after the baby is born; it's vaginal delivery that usually weakens muscles for the long term. When women bear down during the final stages of labor, they stretch the connective tissues that hold up the bladder and urethra. Those organs then sag and weigh on the pelvic floor muscles. Labor and vaginal delivery can also strain the pelvic floor muscles directly and stretch the nerves that feed the muscles, weakening them further.

These problems are greatest when the baby is large or the mother has to push for more than three hours during delivery, says Ingrid Nygaard, M.D., a urogynecologist at the University of Iowa College of Medicine in Iowa City. Those two factors, more than the number of children a woman has, determine which women wind up with stress incontinence.

Tommie Bakun of Crestwood, Illinois, started leaking urine after her second pregnancy. After two more babies, her incontinence became so bad that she had to stop running and playing tennis. She even had to be careful every time she laughed. "You learn to make sure you're always sitting down with your legs crossed before you start joking around," Bakun says.

Some women's postchildbirth incontinence lasts only a few weeks or months, then disappears after the pelvic floor muscles regain their strength and hormone levels return to normal. But when leaking persists longer than six months after childbirth, it's less likely to go away without some kind of intervention.

Incontinence can also strike women who have never been preg-

STAY DRY: CROSS YOUR LEGS

*Y*ou don't have to be humorless until those Kegels start taking effect. Go ahead and let out those laughs, and don't get worried when you think you're about to cough or sneeze. Just cross your legs when it happens and you might stay dry like the Sahara.

Researchers tested what women had been telling them all along and found that women with stress urinary incontinence lost 9½ times less urine when their legs were crossed compared to when they weren't. That could be the difference between having to change clothes after a cough, or just getting rid of a slightly damp pad, says Jan E. Baker, R.N., co-author of this study with Peggy A. Norton, M.D., who is assistant professor in obstetrics and gynecology at the University of Utah School of Medicine in Salt Lake City.

The subtle slip of one knee over the other may boost the power of the pelvic muscles enough to overcome the downward force of the laugh, cough or sneeze, making it more difficult for urine to escape through the urethra.

Crossing the legs is merely a way to manage stress incontinence. To dry up the problem or prevent it in the first place, ask your doctor about Kegel (or pelvic floor) exercises and other forms of managing and treating your incontinence difficulties. The sooner you catch the problem, the more easily it can be managed without surgery.

nant; it occurs most often during strenuous or jarring physical activity such as high-impact aerobics. A recent study of 144 female college varsity athletes found that nearly a third experienced some urine leaks while practicing their sports. The numbers varied according to the kind of sport the athletes participated in: Among gymnasts and basketball players—who presumably performed the highest impact activities—two-thirds were incontinent at least once, while none of the golfers were. The athletic activity did not seem to weaken pelvic floor muscles or cause any general condition of incontinence, says Dr. Nygaard, who conducted the study. "It makes me think that mild incontinence isn't even abnormal," she says. "There may be some threshold of physical activity that over-stresses even the strongest pelvic floor muscles, so that with enough activity, practically anyone would lose urine."

Sexual activity can also trigger incontinence. The likely reasons: the thrusting of a man's penis against his partner's bladder or her pelvic muscle contractions during sex can sometimes push urine out. Karen, a writer living in the Chicago area, leaks urine when she has an orgasm. "It's not pleasant," she says.

Cigarette smokers have a higher-than-average risk of incontinence, perhaps because smoking cuts down the oxygen supply to the tissues supporting the bladder and thus weakens them, says Jill Maura Rabin, M.D., head of urogynecology at Long Island Jewish Medical Center in New Hyde Park, New York. Smoking also makes a woman more prone to coughing, which strains the pelvic floor muscles. Chronic constipation can likewise strain and weaken muscles, leading to incontinence.

Stopping the Leak

The first step in solving a bladder-control problem is getting a proper diagnosis. It's best to consult a urogynecologist or a urologist with expertise in treating female incontinence, since most doctors have not been trained to recognize or treat it. The physician should ask whether urine leaks occur during coughing, sneezing or exercising. She may ask you to cough repeatedly with a full bladder to see if there's leakage. And she may suggest that you keep a record of the number of times you go to the bathroom, the length of time that elapses between trips, the quantity of liquid you drink every day and your activity each time you experience leakage. The physician should also perform a pelvic exam and ask you to contract your pelvic floor muscles to see how strong they are. A urine culture can rule out the possibility that the problem is caused by a bladder infection. A urethral catheter or ultrasound exam may be used to determine whether you are able to empty your bladder completely. (If it turns out that you don't fully void, you could have a condition called overflow incontinence, which may result from defective nerve signals between the bladder and the brain.)

If the diagnosis is mild to moderate stress incontinence, chances are good that the problem can be improved or cured by strengthening

HOW TO KEGEL CORRECTLY

*K*egel exercises can help reduce urinary incontinence. Here's the right way to do them.

Relax your abdomen, thighs and buttocks. Then contract the muscles of the pelvic floor by squeezing them inward and upward as if trying to control a strong urge to urinate. Hold the contraction for up to ten seconds, then release. Do ten long squeezes three times a day.

Chances are your stress incontinence will diminish in two to three months if you do these exercises correctly. Here are three tips to make sure you're on track.

- Concentrate on isolating the right muscles. If you're grimacing, squeezing your legs together or holding in your tummy, you're probably using the wrong muscles.
- Avoid pushing the pelvic floor muscles down as if you're having a bowel movement; it can actually make the problem worse.
- Don't do Kegels while urinating. It's okay to try this once to help figure out where the correct muscles are, but making it a regular practice can cause more problems by training the bladder to empty only partially.

your pelvic floor muscles. The basic exercise is called a Kegel, named after Arnold Kegel, the gynecologist who invented it in 1948. Kegel exercises cured Mary Pieratt of her stress incontinence, though she needed the help of electrical stimulation to learn how to do them correctly. (See "How to Kegel Correctly.") Properly done Kegels can remedy or at least significantly diminish stress incontinence in at least half of women sufferers. To help minimize the problem and keep the bladder from filling too quickly, doctors recommend drinking less coffee, tea, caffeinated soda and alcohol. For the overweight, taking off some pounds can reduce the pressure on the bladder. Dr. Horbach, an incontinence sufferer herself, recently lost 30 pounds and found the problem much less severe.

A physician may also recommend bladder retraining. The idea is to go to the bathroom on a regular schedule, say once every hour. Then, after a week to ten days, increase the time between voiding to an hour and a quarter or an hour and a half. The extra wait forces a woman to contract her pelvic floor muscles and thus improve her ability to be continent.

For those women who pass urine every time they stand up and walk across a room, surgery may offer the only hope. There are two options: anterior repair and bladder suspension. The first involves making tucks in the skin of the top side of the vagina to help support the bladder and urethra. Bladder suspension involves actually lifting the bladder by connecting it to muscles or ligaments higher up in the abdomen. Doctors are now beginning to perform this procedure laparoscopically, with fiber-optic cameras and slender instruments, but incontinence experts warn that the risks and benefits of this technique have not yet been weighed. Studies suggest that bladder suspension is more likely to be successful than anterior repair.

Women whose incontinence results from defective sphincters can have surgery to help correct the problem. Surgeons have effectively strengthened sphincters by injecting collagen into the juncture between the bladder and the urethra, which increases the external pressure on the urethra and helps keep it closed.

Whatever approach a woman takes, she may find that she does not become 100 percent accident-free. She still may leak a little, for example, when she coughs with a full bladder. But at least she can stop sitting in a chair with her legs crossed and return to an active life.

For help in locating a physician who specializes in treating incontinence, contact Help for Incontinent People (HIP) at P.O. Box 544, Union, SC 29379; or call 1-800-BLADDER. For answers to questions about incontinence or for more information, contact HIP or the Simon Foundation for Continence, P.O. Box 835, Wilmette, IL 60091; or call 1-800-23-SIMON.

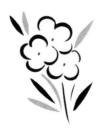

Thyroid Disease: A Woman's Guide

Feeling cold or run-down—or hot and shaky—may signal an out-of-kilter thyroid.

Two years ago, Heidi Bowman of North Canton, Ohio, wasn't feeling like her old energetic self. She needed all the zip she could muster to keep up with her three boys, but instead she felt sluggish and tired, no matter how much sleep she got. Then her periods became irregular and she noticed her short-term memory was fading. Because her symptoms were so vague, her doctor tested her for such diverse illnesses as Lyme disease, mononucleosis and anemia. When these tests proved negative, the doctor homed in on her thyroid. It was slightly underactive.

Doctors have long known that women over age 40 are disproportionately affected by disorders of the thyroid, a small, butterfly-shaped gland nestled in the middle of the neck. Now, thanks to sensitive diagnostic blood tests, the earliest stages of these problems are being recognized in many younger women. Early detection and treatment can prevent these disorders from damaging the gland and other organs and can alleviate fertility problems and improve a woman's overall health and well-being.

Too Much Hormone—Or Not Enough

The thyroid regulates metabolism and influences the functioning of the heart, brain, liver, kidneys and skin. Its workings are directed by the pituitary gland via a complex hormonal signaling system. The pituitary gland produces thyroid-stimulating hormone (TSH), which alerts the thyroid to release two body-regulating hormones, thyroxine (T4) and triodithyronine (T3). In roughly one in eight women, at some time during their lives, a malfunctioning autoimmune system disrupts the signals between the two glands. For unknown reasons (genetics appears to play a role, and estrogen may too), the body produces antibodies that attack the thyroid. Usually the result is an underproduction of hormones, or *hypo*thyroidism, which causes the pituitary gland to send out too much TSH. Less frequently, it's an overproduction of T4 and T3, or *hyper*thyroidism, which suppresses TSH output by the pituitary gland. (The improved thyroid tests detect the slightest elevation or decline of TSH levels in the bloodstream.)

Five to seven million people have hypothyroidism, a disorder that affects women five to eight times more often than men. In roughly half of these cases, those afflicted may not even suspect a problem because the symptoms are subtle and often develop gradually. Women who do feel symptoms may attribute their body slowdown to stress, overwork or aging. And doctors may miss the early stages of disease because it's not common practice to assess thyroid function in young women.

One million to two and a half million Americans have hyperthyroidism, which is five to ten times more common in women than in men. Hyperthyroidism is often easier to diagnose than hypothyroidism because the symptoms, such as heart palpitations, tremors and heat sensitivity, tend to be more alarming and distinct, says Susan Burke, M.D., an endocrinologist affiliated with Northwestern University Medical School in Chicago.

Left untreated, thyroid diseases can cause a variety of symptoms (see "Recognizing Thyroid Trouble"). They can also lead to more serious disorders. "Hyperthyroidism can lead to muscle weakness, decreased bone mass and cardiac problems," says Dr. Burke, "and hypothyroidism can cause depression."

Thyroid disorders also have a major influence on reproductive functioning: They can alter hormone levels, disrupt menstrual cycles and impair fertility, according to Stanley Feld, M.D., president of the American Association of Clinical Endocrinologists. Close monitoring of TSH levels and treatment can alleviate many of these problems and help a woman to successfully conceive and deliver a child, says Dr. Feld.

After delivery, up to 10 percent of women experience postpartum thyroiditis—a transient, usually mild inflammation of the thyroid

RECOGNIZING THYROID TROUBLE

*B*ody clues to hypo- and hyperthyroidism may be very subtle. Here are the most common symptoms for each disorder.

Hypothyroidism	Hyperthyroidism
Fatigue	Nervousness
Loss of interest and/or pleasure	Irritability
Forgetfulness	Sleeping difficulties
Dry, coarse hair	Bulging eyes
Loss of lateral eyebrow hair	Unblinking stare
Puffy face and eyes	Thyroid enlargement
Thyroid enlargement	(called a goiter)
(called a goiter)	Rapid heartbeat
Dry skin	Increased sweating
Cold intolerance	Heat intolerance
Weight gain	Unexplained weight loss
Heavy menstrual periods	Light, infrequent menstrual
Constipation	periods
Brittle nails	Warm, moist palms
Slow heartbeat	Fine tremor of fingers

caused by pregnancy-related changes in the immune system. These fluctuations in thyroid functioning can trigger symptoms that can easily be confused with normal postpartum changes. "If you experience any subtle symptoms consistent with thyroid disease after delivery, ask your doctor to perform one of the new, more sensitive TSH tests," says Dr. Burke.

Testing and Diagnosis

Although endocrinologists have been able to measure TSH levels for the past 15 years, the new, more sensitive tests now make it possible for doctors to accurately detect mild or subclinical disease. The so-called sensitive TSH test is 10 to 100 times more sensitive than the standard test, and the newer ultrasensitive TSH test is 10 times more sensitive than that, says Boston endocrinologist Reed Larsen, M.D., president of the American Thyroid Association. The tests cost anywhere from $40 to $90, according to a survey by the Thyroid Foundation of America. If the TSH test is abnormal, other tests that measure T3 and T4 levels may be necessary.

If you're diagnosed with an overt thyroid disorder, you'll need treatment to clear up your symptoms and prevent more serious health problems. But doctors are also recognizing that women with subclinical hypothyroidism (and, to a lesser degree, hyperthyroidism) also need to be followed closely and possibly treated, even if they don't have any symptoms. The reason: Each year, 5 to 20 percent of women with subclinical hypothyroidism go on to develop the full-blown disorder.

"Women often aren't aware that they have been suffering from the effects of a thyroid problem until they've been treated and they see an improvement in their energy level and quality of life," notes H. Jack Baskin, M.D., founder of the Florida Thyroid and Endocrine Clinic in Orlando. "In addition, treatment of subclinical hypothyroidism can significantly reduce cholesterol levels and restore fertility."

Treatment of hypothyroidism consists of thyroid hormone replacement therapy—a pill a day for life. Doctors prescribe a synthetic T4 and recommend brand names such as Levothroid, Levoxine and Synthroid over generics. A year's supply of pills costs between $30 and $100. Once treatment starts, close monitoring is advised, as the body's requirement for thyroid hormone fluctuates. Even a dose that's just 10 percent too high can harm health by increasing the risk of osteoporosis and heart disease, says Dr. Baskin. The new TSH tests provide doctors with an accurate, easy means of annually determining the body's requirement for replacement thyroid hormone. (During your first year of treatment, your doctor may want to check your TSH levels every couple of months to find the right dosage.)

Most people diagnosed with hyperthyroidism are treated with radioactive iodine therapy, which disables the thyroid gland and halts thyroid hormone production completely within three to six months. This treatment is considered safe and free of long-term side effects or complications. Surgery to remove the gland—once standard treatment—is now rarely performed.

Over 40? Get Tested. Under 40? Ditto.

Given the prevalence of thyroid disease among women, the American Association of Clinical Endocrinologists is now calling for all women over 40 to be screened annually with a sensitive or ultra-sensitive hormone test to identify subclinical hypothyroidism. But Dr. Baskin advocates sensitive hormone tests every year or two for women in their twenties and thirties because he sees so many female patients with subtle thyroid disease.

Heidi Bowman is thankful that her disease was caught early. "All I have to do is take a pill each morning and have my TSH measured periodically to make sure I'm receiving the right dose," she says. "It's inexpensive and convenient—and I have my old pep back."

For more information on thyroid disorders or referrals for doctors in your area, contact the Thyroid Society for Education and Research, 7515 South Main Street, Suite 545, Houston, TX 77030; 1-800-THYROID.

Beat the "Big Three"

Women, too, are vulnerable to heart disease, high blood pressure and stroke. But you can protect yourself.

*M*ore and more American women are taking control of their health—learning about their bodies, questioning the quality of their health care, demanding information about their unique health concerns. And as more and more women are discovering, "male" maladies like heart disease, high blood pressure and stroke affect women as well.

But there's a lot you can do to safeguard your health and quality of life—right now. Here's how to thwart the "Big Three" and gear up for a disease-free future.

DON'T FORGET THE BASICS

*H*ere are five more ways you can reduce your risk of developing heart disease, hypertension and cancer.

Stop smoking. Not only does smoking top the list of risk factors for a number of cancers, it plays a huge role in raising blood pressure and increasing heart disease risk, too. Smoking a single cigarette raises blood pressure for up to an hour, which translates into day-long hypertension for pack-a-day puffers.

It's *never* too late to kick the habit. After 1 year smoke-free, your heart disease risk will decrease by 50 percent, and after 10 to 15 years, your risk for early death will be about the same as a nonsmoker's. For information on quitting for good, call the American Lung Association at 1-800-LUNG-USA.

If you're a nonsmoker, do your best to avoid exposure to tobacco smoke. Living with someone who smokes or working eight hours a day in a smoky environment can raise your cancer risk, possibly by 50 percent.

Go easy on alcohol. Folks who drink three or more alcoholic beverages a day are more likely to develop high blood pressure than those who drink less. And heavy drinking greatly increases the risk of cancers of the mouth, throat and liver.

Don't think you have to give up an occasional libation, however: Some studies have shown that drinking 1 to 2 ounces of hard liquor, 8 ounces of wine or 12 ounces of beer daily can raise levels of "good" high-density lipoprotein (HDL) cholesterol. But it's still best to limit

Five Ways to Protect Your Heart

Are you intimidated by heart disease? It's understandable—but you shouldn't be. While it's the number one killer of American women (and men), you really can prevent heart disease from shortening your life. Here's how.

Get annual checkups. One of the best ways to learn whether your heart's at risk is to have your doctor check your blood pressure and cholesterol levels every year. If you have high blood pressure or high levels of low-density lipoprotein (LDL) cholesterol (the kind that clogs arteries) and low levels of high-density lipoprotein (HDL) cholesterol (the kind that puts the brakes on LDL), you're more likely to develop your intake because excessive drinking raises *total* cholesterol, which can lead to heart problems.

Take a walk. Regular aerobic exercise, such as 20 to 30 minutes of brisk walking three or four times a week, can lower existing high blood pressure (or prevent it from occurring) and help change your cholesterol profile, leading to a reduced risk of heart disease. What's more, some experts believe there's a positive link between regular exercise and cancer prevention. Talk to your doctor before you begin exercising and don't change your intake of medication unless she tells you to do so.

Trim down. Studies have linked obesity (being 20 percent or more overweight) with increased risk of colon, prostate and gallbladder cancers. What's more, the heavier you are, the harder your heart must work to pump blood through your body, and this extra effort is likely to increase your blood pressure.

The safest way to lose any extra weight is to adopt a program of exercise and to modify your diet (see below). Be sure to consult your physician first, however.

Eat wisely. The less fat you eat, the less fat will clog your arteries and put you at risk for heart disease, stroke and hypertension. What's more, the National Cancer Institute reports that dietary factors probably account for up to 35 percent of all cancers. So ferret fatty foods (such as red meat, eggs and whole dairy products) from your diet and opt for whole grains, vegetables, fruits and fish instead.

cardiovascular diseases, which could lead to heart attack or stroke.

Lower your pressure. High blood pressure puts extra strain on your heart and arteries, and, ultimately, can provoke a heart attack. (See below for tips on keeping your blood pressure reading in a healthy range.)

Consider aspirin. Aspirin helps prevent blood from clotting and thereby protects against the most common cause of heart attacks: blockages in the arteries. William P. Castelli, M.D., medical director of the Framingham Heart Study in Framingham, Massachusetts, says that taking regular doses of aspirin is probably a good idea if the following are true:

- You've already had a heart attack.
- You have high blood pressure.
- You have a high level of cholesterol in your bloodstream.
- You're diabetic.

George Sopko, M.D., a cardiologist at the National Heart, Lung and Blood Institute in Bethesda, Maryland, recommends taking no more than 81 milligrams of aspirin daily. (Higher doses may lead to irritation of the stomach lining.) But consult your doctor before you begin taking regular doses of aspirin.

Be happy. A happy heart's more likely to be a healthy one. In fact, according to many experts, being involved in loving relationships is a better heart helper than ditching the salt shaker and switching from regular coffee to decaf. Another way to reduce your risk of heart problems is to tame the tension in your life. A bonus: Eliminating stress won't only make you happier and healthier, it'll help keep your immune system strong, too.

Consider HRT. If you're a postmenopausal woman, hormone replacement therapy could be an important means of protecting your heart. Estrogen elevates HDL levels and decreases LDL levels, in addition to lowering your blood pressure and helping you maintain a healthy weight—which may be why it lowers the incidence of heart disease among women.

One word of warning, however: Hormone therapy may slightly increase your risk of developing breast cancer, so steer clear of this treatment if you're already at risk for this disease. Also, discuss your options for cancer screening programs and heart disease treatments with your physician.

Lower Your Blood Pressure

The bad news: Left untreated, high blood pressure (hypertension) will dramatically increase your chances of suffering a stroke or heart attack or dying of congestive heart failure. High blood pressure can also contribute to kidney disease and problems with eyesight, memory and even sexual performance.

The good news: Hypertension is not only treatable, it's preventable.

Healthy blood pressure for most people at age 60 is 130/90, while any reading that consistently hits 140/90 or higher is considered risky, no matter what your age. Note that the operative word here is *consistently*. Blood pressure fluctuates throughout the day depending on your activity and stress levels, which is perfectly normal. The problems arise when your pressure increases and then remains elevated. Here are four ways to keep that from happening.

Check your BP regularly. The symptoms of high blood pressure can be subtle, so you may not know if you have it unless you get your pressure checked. To be sure yours is within the healthy range, have your doctor take your blood pressure reading annually. Experts say that this simple act could save 15,000 lives every year.

Lower your salt intake. The chloride in sodium chloride, better known as table salt, is a major cause of high blood pressure. To keep your salt intake low, don't use salt when cooking and replace the white stuff in your salt shaker with a no-salt blend of herbs and spices. Also, choose low-salt or no-salt versions of processed foods, such as soups, lunch meats and cheeses.

Pack away potassium. Not getting enough potassium may substantially increase your risk of getting hypertension as well as worsen existing high blood pressure. "Studies suggest, though, that when you get the right amount of potassium, the positive change in blood pressure may lead to a reduction in risk of stroke," says G. Gopal Krishna, M.D., a practitioner at Central Coast Nephrology in Salinas, California. To pump up your potassium intake, eat plenty of bananas, potatoes, broccoli, tomatoes and orange juice.

Learn to relax. When you're feeling anxious, angry or depressed, try using stress-management techniques to help you relax. Methods such as these can reduce mild hypertension and effectively counteract increases in blood pressure.

Cancer-Proof Your Body

In a recent survey, 200 American doctors and scientists on the front lines of cancer research and treatment were asked how people can reduce their cancer risk. Half of the experts agreed that 50 to 70 percent of all cancers could be prevented with the right lifestyle modifications. So take note of the following doctor-recommended anti-cancer actions and start making changes—today.

Get tested. Regular cancer screenings and self-exams won't help prevent cancer, but they *will* help you detect it at an early, possibly curable stage. Look into your family's history of cancer, and talk with your physician about developing a screening program that's appropriate for you.

Screen out the sun. Essentially, all of the 500,000-plus annual cases of non-melanoma skin cancer are caused by overexposure to sunlight, says Paul F. Engstrom, M.D., senior vice-president of the Fox Chase Cancer Center in Philadelphia. Short of permanently staying indoors, your best bet is to keep your skin covered with sunscreen that has a sun protection factor of at least 15 and guards against both UVA and UVB rays.

Think positively. Recent studies show that reducing stress can bring about measurable changes in immune function. "It's hard to prove scientifically that a positive outlook can help prevent cancer," says Peter Greenwald, M.D., of the National Cancer Institute headquarters in Bethesda, Maryland. "But many people—doctors included—have a feeling that people with a positive attitude may smoke less and have better eating habits." And it's lifestyle factors such as these that can keep cancer out of the picture.

Consider your environment. Many experts rate environmental factors amazingly low in importance as a cause of cancer, but there is some controversy in this area. Experts disagree on whether or not it's best to avoid exposure to radon (a gas that leaches through the ground into some homes) and electromagnetic fields (produced by high-tension wires, electric blankets and computer screens).

To be on the safe side, you can try to avoid these factors, but more important is whether or not your job regularly exposes you to hazardous chemicals. There's solid evidence linking certain industrial agents such as nickel, chromate, asbestos and vinyl chloride to increased cancer risks. If your job exposes you to any of these agents, find out what precautions your company is taking to protect you from overexposure.

How Women Can Dodge Diabetes

Making a few lifestyle changes can actually help women avert this potentially debilitating disorder.

Is your lifestyle so inactive that cleaning the house is an indoor sport and running for the bus an Olympic event? You could be putting yourself at risk for diabetes, and it could show up between age 30 and 45.

More than seven million American women have diabetes, about the same number as men. Five to 10 percent have Type I, or insulin-dependent, diabetes, an inherited disease in which the immune system attacks the pancreas and destroys its ability to make insulin, the hormone that transports sugar from food to your body's cells. Type I usually appears sometime in childhood or adolescence, but it also occurs in adults.

The remaining 90 to 95 percent have Type II, or non-insulin-dependent, diabetes, a disease in which the body cannot use all the insulin it produces. Type II has genetic roots, but it's often triggered in women by too much testosterone, the male sex hormone, or by a sedentary lifestyle.

Testosterone is not a factor in the development of Type II diabetes in men, studies indicate, but high levels of it seem to double or even triple the risk among women. What's more, a study of 165 women at the University of Texas Health Sciences Center in San Antonio revealed that the more testosterone a woman's body produces, the more likely she is to develop diabetes.

At least half of the women with Type II diabetes don't know they have it, experts say. This is because until the disease explodes with its complications—heart disease, stroke, blindness or kidney failure— signs of diabetes are frequently subtle. Also, some blood tests used to identify the disease frequently fail to detect it.

This failure can be dangerous, since a woman with diabetes has 6 times the risk of heart attack as a woman who does not have it. She also has nearly 20 times the risk of kidney failure, nearly 5 times the risk of stroke and 3 times the risk of death; she is also a prime candidate for both blindness and the nerve damage that can lead to amputation.

Famine in the Midst of Plenty

Diabetes is a disease that forces your body to starve when it's full of food.

Normally your body takes last night's dinner or this morning's breakfast and turns it into a sugar called glucose. Then it dumps the glucose into your blood, where it teams up with insulin secreted by your pancreas. The insulin carries glucose into your muscles and organs, where it provides the energy for everything you do.

A drop in available insulin or the body's resistance to using that insulin can cause metabolic mayhem. With diabetes, glucose builds up in the bloodstream because it's unable to gain admission to muscles and organs. It wears on the heart, kidneys and eyes and then it flows into the bladder and passes out of the body—leaving behind damaged organs starved for fuel.

Left too long in this situation, the body powers down: In both Type I and Type II diabetes, excessive hunger, thirst, fatigue and urination are all cries for help that—left unheeded—can lead to lethargy, coma and death.

Good News: Prevention Is Possible

Both forms of diabetes can be treated with a smorgasbord of custom-tailored diets, exercise, insulin injections and other medications.

"MY GENERATION IS
THE FIRST TO SURVIVE"

*K*ate Sullivan is a mother and part-time public affairs officer for the National Kidney Foundation in Philadelphia. She has lived with Type I (insulin-dependent) diabetes since she was born. This is her story.

My mother started giving me the responsibility for handling the disease when I was about eight years old. I remember the first time that I tried to give myself an insulin shot. I really had to psych myself into it. And this was just injecting into the top of my leg, which isn't really a big deal. But it was very difficult.

Long before blood testing and even before they came up with those handy little dipsticks for urine testing, we used a chemistry set with little glass test tubes and these little tablets that would dissolve in water. They came in little foil packets. You had to put so many drops of urine and so many drops of water into the test tube, then put the little pill in and watch the whole thing fizz up and watch for what color it turned. I also had a metal needle that attached to a glass syringe which came apart. Every morning we boiled all three parts inside a strainer which was inside a saucepan on the stove.

What kept me doing it?

We had a neighbor who lived around the corner who had diabetes. He was minus a foot. And through the years gangrene started to claim parts of his leg. So every time I would see him, he would have less of one leg. And my mother kept saying, "Well, that's a diabetic just like you." You want to talk about keeping a little kid in line?

I mean, I want to live. I don't want to forever be the kid with her nose pressed up against the candy store window looking at the kids inside.

It's only as I've become an adult and looked back on this that I realize that my generation is really the first generation to survive—to get not only to adulthood but to start to get into some of the problems that the middle-age and aging populations normally face. Before, doctors never had to worry about diabetes and heart disease because diabetics never got old.

So it's our observations and our experiences that are going to form the body of information for the generation that comes behind us. It's scary because there's no blueprint. On the other hand, thank God I'm in this generation and not the one before it.

ARE YOU AT RISK?

*D*iabetes runs in families, but no one has been able to figure out how or why.

The problem is the complexity of the disease and its genetic connections. "It doesn't seem to be a single gene disease," explains Maureen Harris, M.D., Ph.D., director of the National Diabetes Data Group at the National Institutes of Health in Washington, D.C. "It may be that there's more than one gene involved, or it may be that there's an interaction with the environment."

In any case, studies show that the children of a mother or father with Type I, or insulin-dependent, diabetes have about a 2 to 5 percent risk of developing the disease. The children of a parent with Type II, or non-insulin-dependent, diabetes have about a 10 to 15 percent chance.

There's no known way to prevent the onset of Type I if it is written on your genetic program, but the risk of Type II diabetes can be reduced simply by maintaining your ideal weight, eating a low-fat diet and getting plenty of exercise.

But these treatment strategies sometimes fail to prevent the degenerative problems that go with diabetes.

That's why prevention is so important, says Maureen Harris, M.D., Ph.D., director of the National Diabetes Data Group at the National Institutes of Health in Washington, D.C. Here's what you can do.

Get an early warning. Type II diabetes doesn't emerge as a full-blown problem overnight, says Wendy Kohrt, Ph.D., research assistant professor of medicine at Washington University in St. Louis. It generally evolves over a period of years and can be detected in its earliest stages by a blood test that reveals whether your body is beginning to have trouble using insulin.

"Most clinicians don't measure insulin," explains Dr. Kohrt. "They measure glucose. And they're not concerned until it's over 140 (milligrams per deciliter)." But she says that more than 50 percent of those diagnosed with diabetes have fasting blood sugar levels around 100 to 120 milligrams.

Lose weight. "The higher your weight, the higher your risk of diabetes," explains Richard Hamman, M.D., Ph.D., professor of preventive medicine at the University of Colorado School of Medicine in Boulder.

You especially need to lose weight if your body is shaped like an apple—thick in the middle, he adds. Why? Because "the fat in that region is different from other fat in two respects. First, it's metabolically more active, which means it's stored and mobilized more readily," says Dr. Kohrt. Second, that fat is in an area drained by a major vein that picks up the fat's metabolic by-products and takes them to the liver. There they give the liver a false message—that fat is being mobilized because the body is starving. But the liver doesn't know the message is false, so it responds by churning out an emergency ration of glucose into the bloodstream.

"That begins a vicious cycle that just keeps going," says Dr. Kohrt. More glucose in the blood makes the pancreas dump in more insulin. More insulin causes the liver to generate more glucose. More glucose makes the pancreas dump more insulin. Eventually, the whole system breaks down, says Dr. Kohrt. Your body will either shut down insulin production or the muscles and organs will refuse to accept it. Either way, you have diabetes.

To figure out whether you fall into this high-risk group, "take a tape measure and move it up and down between waist and hip," says Dr. Hamman. "Then use the smallest waist and largest hip measures to figure the waist/hip ratio." Divide the hip measurement into the waist measurement and see what you get.

In women the waist/hip ratio should be about 0.8. If you have a 1 or a 1.1, that suggests you have a type of fat that predisposes you to diabetes, says Dr. Hamman.

Cut dietary fat. As you start to lose weight, pay particular attention to the amount of fat in your diet, says Dr. Hamman. That's because, independently of its effect on weight, dietary fat seems to increase the risk of diabetes.

Doctors and other experts recommend that you limit your daily diet to less than 30 percent of calories from fat. Some experts advise cutting back on fat even more, to 25 percent of calories from fat. You can aim for this by limiting your intake of meat, always removing skin from poultry, avoiding processed foods and drinking low-fat milk. (For more tips on following a low-fat lifestyle, see page 170.)

Get moving. "Women who are sedentary probably have a 25 to 40 percent increased risk of diabetes compared to women who are more active at the same weight," Dr. Hamman says.

"Active is walking down to the corner grocery rather than getting in your car to drive," Dr. Kohrt says. "It's taking the dog for a one- or two-mile walk instead of putting him outside in a fenced-in yard. It's going up three or four flights of steps rather than taking elevators." And it's doing these things day in and day out.

The result? "If you have a 180-pound woman who loses weight and maintains it, decreases her dietary fat and increases her physical activity, I suspect she would cut her diabetes risk fivefold," says Dr. Hamman.

Thwarting Diabetes during Pregnancy

Pregnancy is a time of great adjustment for a woman and her body. Raging hormones cause nausea, fatigue, physical change and an abundance of emotions—all part of a healthy, normal pregnancy. But these same hormones can trigger diabetes in a woman who has never before been diabetic—a condition known as gestational diabetes.

Women who develop gestational diabetes have different risks than women with diabetes who become pregnant. Those who develop diabetes during pregnancy tend to have chubbier babies and a higher incidence of unexplained stillbirths. They are also at greater risk for developing the pregnancy-related high blood pressure known as preeclampsia.

Women with diabetes who become pregnant, on the other hand, tend to have smaller babies. They have a greater risk of birth defects and of maternal and fetal death.

Here are some ways to minimize the chances of developing gestational diabetes, or reduce its effects.

Eat for one. "The woman who starts to gain a lot of weight is more inclined to develop gestational diabetes," says Yvonne S. Thornton, M.D., professor of clinical obstetrics and gynecology at Columbia

University College of Physicians and Surgeons in New York City, and director of perinatal diagnostic testing at Morristown Memorial Hospital in New Jersey. Despite the old story about eating for two, you really need only 300 extra calories a day through the second trimester and 500 in the third.

Eat beans. Studies indicate that folic acid, a nutrient that all women need, may prevent the neural tube defects that can occur when diabetes is uncontrolled, says Helen Kay, M.D., a specialist in maternal/fetal medicine and associate professor of obstetrics and gynecology at Duke University in Durham, North Carolina. (Researchers have found that folic acid helps prevent the overall incidence of spinal defects in the fetus, whether or not the woman has diabetes.) Beans are a good source of folic acid. A half-cup of red beans, pinto beans, mung beans, navy beans, black beans or lima beans will give you more than half of the Recommended Dietary Allowance for pregnant women (400 micrograms a day).

Get tested. Ask your obstetrician to test you for diabetes between the 24th and 28th weeks of pregnancy, says Dr. Kay. Usually, you'll be asked to drink a glucose solution that tastes like "a flat cola," then you'll be given a blood test to measure glucose levels an hour later. If that test shows high levels of glucose, you'll be asked to come back for a second test that measures glucose levels over a three-hour period.

If your glucose level is high, your doctor or nutritionist will probably prescribe the American Diabetes Association diet in an attempt to control it, says Dr. Thornton. "If your blood sugar remains high, you'll have to get insulin injections three or four times a day and follow the diet."

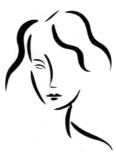

Tired of Being Tired?

You're up with the sun. And by 7:00 P.M., you're down for the count. If you're drop-dead exhausted, try these rejuvenating tactics.

The alarm goes off at 6:00 A.M. You snuggle with your mate for a moment, push the dog off the bed and reach for your moccasins.

You get breakfast for the kids, throw a load in the washer, get dressed, drop the cat at the vet, pick up the dry cleaning and get yourself to work. And it's only 9:00 A.M.

Then you work like a dog trying to meet the deadlines and responsibilities of your job.

It's almost a relief when you stuff a little of the work into your briefcase at 6:00 P.M., grab your keys and head for home.

Once there, of course, life's a breeze. You make dinner, supervise homework, get the kids to bed and fold the laundry. Then, with pillows propped behind you and a cup of hot tea at your side, you pull out the work you brought home from the office.

Why Women Are So Bushed

Women have always worked hard. But today, doctors say, women are exhausted. Married or single, with or without kids, working in an office, a laundry or at home, it seems as true as ever that a woman's work is never done.

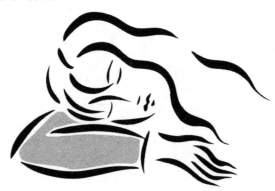

The result is that fatigue is one of the top ten complaints in doctors' offices across the country.

That's not to say that the deadening fatigue of which women are complaining can't be caused by physical ailments. It can. Fatigue is a side effect of almost every disease and condition known to woman. It can be caused by pregnancy, menopause, an approaching period, overweight, flu, anemia, mononucleosis, cancer, a low-grade urinary tract infection, a vaginal infection, diabetes, hypoglycemia, depression, fibromyalgia, the common cold, smoking, stress or just having your thyroid out of whack.

It can also be caused by drugs. Antihistamines, tranquilizers, muscle relaxants, sedatives, narcotics, birth control pills, heart medications and pain relievers can all cause fatigue.

Then there is chronic fatigue syndrome, which is something completely different. Some doctors believe it's caused by some kind of malfunction in the immune system.

But when a woman shows up in a doctor's office with fatigue as her chief complaint, the problem is not usually illness or medication.

"I think that people feel chronically tired for a very simple reason," says fatigue researcher Anthony Komaroff, M.D., professor of medicine at Harvard Medical School. "They're working long, hard hours."

The work week in the United States has been steadily increasing since the mid-1960s, says Dr. Komaroff, particularly for women. It's one of the most important phenomena of our time, he adds. Yet it's a cultural trend that most Americans haven't yet recognized.

Why? They're too busy working.

The Incomplete Revolution

Why are women working so hard? The problem for most women is that they're caught between social revolutions, experts agree. While one social revolution has expanded women's roles to provide increased career opportunities, a second, hoped-for social revolution— that of increased men's roles in the family—hasn't come to fruition.

In the 1993 National Study of the Changing Workforce, researchers at the Families and Work Institute, a New York City-based think tank, surveyed 3,000 working Americans and found that while men were spending more time working in the home than their fathers, women were still working twice as many hours as men at home. The overwhelming majority of women (81 percent) did most of the shopping and cooking, 78 percent did the bulk of the cleaning, 71 percent assumed primary responsibility for child care, and 63 percent took charge of the check-writing and bill-paying.

Most men (91 percent) did the household repairs, and 35 percent of men did most of the check-writing. Eighteen percent did the shopping, 15 percent did most of the cooking, 7 percent did the cleaning, and 5 percent took responsibility for child care.

"Men think they're doing more, but when you compare what they say they're doing with what their wives say they're doing, there's a 50-point spread," says Dana Friedman, Ed.D., co-president of the Families and Work Institute and one of the researchers who conducted the study.

Blame the Economy, Too

A second reason women are working so hard is that men's failure to assume 50-50 responsibility for home, hearth and kids is taking place against a backdrop of what newspapers frequently label "economic uncertainty."

Translation: People are terrified they'll lose their jobs.

In the Changing Workforce study, researchers found that 42 percent of those surveyed worked in companies that had downsized or made permanent cutbacks in the workforce during the previous year. Twenty-eight percent witnessed cutbacks in the number of managers in their workplace, 24 percent saw a change in their company's top leadership, and 18 percent were affected by a merger or acquisition.

In the wake of this much corporate turbulence, it's not surprising that nearly 35 percent of those surveyed expected to temporarily or permanently lose their jobs in the near future.

Nor is it surprising to learn that in this "lean and mean" environment, women are working their hearts out.

Eighty percent say that their workplaces require working very hard,

---

THE PERFECT PICK-ME-UP

*L*ow-fat, high-carb foods such as cereals and breads, pasta, potatoes, vegetables and fruit are most likely to add energy to your day, nutritionists say. But an excellent choice for a quick pickup during that 4:00 P.M. energy sag would be one of the following fruits.

- 1 medium banana
- 1 orange
- ¼ cup raisins
- 5 dates, dried or fresh
- ¼ honeydew melon
- ½ medium cantaloupe
- 3 medium apricots, fresh, canned or dried
- ½ medium apple
- 2 figs, dried or fresh

---

65 percent say that they're required to work very fast, 43 percent say that they have an excessive amount of work, and 27 percent say that there's not enough time scheduled for the amount of work allotted.

The result? Married or not, moms or not, 42 percent of working women surveyed said they usually feel used up at the end of the workday. And 40 percent of all employees said they wake up tired almost every morning.

Energizing (and Empowering) Advice

Neither men nor corporations are likely to change overnight. So how do you fight fatigue in the 1990s? Here's what experts say.

Prioritize. "Most of us are still assuming the traditional responsibilities that society says a 'real' woman does," says Claire Etaugh, Ph.D., professor of psychology and dean of the College of Liberal Arts and Sciences at Bradley University in Peoria, Illinois. But just because our moms baked apple pies, had hot chocolate waiting after school and kept the toilet bowl sparkling doesn't mean that we should—especially not in a world where an attorney who works 40 hours a week is considered a part-timer.

"There are too many 'shoulds' in our lives," says Dr. Etaugh. "You have to decide what's most important, set priorities and then—whether it's cleaning, family, friendships or career—let the rest go."

Drop the guilt. If not fulfilling your own image of a perfect wife, mom, worker or housekeeper makes you feel guilty, see a therapist, adds Dr. Etaugh. Otherwise, feeling guilty over not baking your son's favorite cherry pie could leave you feeling just as exhausted as if you'd taken the time to make it.

Learn to manage your time. Most working women—particularly working mothers—are highly efficient at managing their time. But it always helps to have someone else look at your workload, both at home and at work, with a critical eye. There's a good chance that somewhere, somehow, there's a more efficient—that is, less fatiguing—way to get things done.

To find a local workshop or seminar on time management, call a local college, YWCA or chamber of commerce and ask if they know of any in the area. You should also check the Yellow Pages of your telephone directory and keep an eye out for ads in women's business magazines.

Try to talk to prospective workshop leaders on the phone before you sign up, advises Dr. Etaugh. Outline the demands on your life and ask how they'll address them.

Do two things at once. Become an expert at figuring out how to do more than one thing at a time, says Dr. Etaugh. Hang an extra cleaning brush on the shower caddy and scrub down the walls when you shower. Fold laundry while you listen to a theme your child has written for tomorrow's class.

Use the phone. Bank by phone. Pay by phone. Use direct-mail catalogs and 800 numbers to shop at home. Order gifts by phone—then have them wrapped and sent, says Dr. Etaugh.

Take control of your worklife. "Probably the most tiring situation is to have responsibility without authority in the workplace," says Susan Schenkel, Ph.D., Cambridge, Massachusetts, psychologist and author of Giving Away Success: Why Women Get Stuck and What to Do about It. "It makes things difficult, unpleasant and exhausting. And it's a big workplace issue for a lot of women," she says.

Moving up the corporate ladder—or even sideways—into a different job is one answer, as is looking for another job or quitting and starting your own business. Either way, says Dr. Schenkel, taking control of what you do and when you do it is a big energy booster.

Talk to your boss. If you're finding more and more work on your desk, Dr. Etaugh says, talk to your supervisor and try to work out a more manageable workload.

Check the parking lot. To avoid taking the kind of job in which a 60-hour week is the norm, cruise through the parking lot of any company you're thinking of working for at about 6:00 A.M. or 6:00 P.M. during the week, suggests Dr. Friedman. Count the number of cars. If there are one or two, no problem. But if the lot is a quarter full, there's a good chance that this is a corporation that pushes its people to the wall.

Exercise. "Fatigue is a big problem for me," says Dr. Schenkel. "That's why I spend a considerable amount of time working out. I do sit-ups and stretches every morning. And I try to spend about 25 minutes a day on the exercise bike. Then every other day I try to walk for anywhere from 40 minutes to an hour."

Besides keeping your energy levels up on a long-term basis, exercise can also energize you on the spot, doctors agree. In a study at California State University, for example, researchers compared the energy levels of a group of volunteers who took a ten-minute walk and a group who ate candy instead. The researchers found that the walkers increased their energy more than the munchers, and the effects of walking lasted much longer than those of munching—up to two hours.

Energize your diet. "Another factor that makes a lot of women tired is that they have poor nutrition," says Dr. Schenkel. Nutrition experts suggest that a high-energy diet is one that's high in complex carbohydrates like those found in grains, beans, pasta and most baked goods, with less than 25 percent of its calories coming from fatty foods. And if you really must lose weight, keep your energy levels up by keeping your calorie intake above 1,000 a day.

Get help. If you can afford it, hire someone to clean the house, mow the lawn and babysit the kids, and have the pizza delivered.

The Alternative Route

Since so many illnesses can cause an overwhelming sense of fatigue, check with your family doctor whenever you feel exhausted for more than a few weeks.

But if your doctor gives you a clean bill of health even when you're still exhausted, think about consulting a professional who practices alternative medicine, says Dr. Schenkel.

"If you go to your average doctor and tell him that you're tired and he doesn't find anything interesting on his tests, he will say, 'You need to reduce your stress, and God be with you, Madam,' " she says. But a physician who practices alternative medicine will take the fact that you're tired as important information. Ask your doctor to refer you to someone who practices this kind of medicine.

For instance, Dr. Schenkel says, "in oriental medicine, doctors organize their whole medical system around energy—around the concept of *chi*. So someone who practices oriental medicine will be curious about where in your body the *chi* is blocked, and they'll help you try to unblock it," possibly with acupuncture, herbs and exercise.

Who knows? says Dr. Schenkel. Maybe an hour or two of slow, flowing movements of the Chinese exercise tai chi chuan every week is all you need to re-energize.

Sleep Better, Feel Better

You've suffered through the late-night infomercials and you're still wide-awake. These hints can help you drop off.

Judith Evnen Benson, a therapist from LaVista, Nebraska, knows that if she gets out of bed and takes more than 30 steps, she'll be awake the rest of the night. Of course, her 16-month-old son doesn't know that, so occasionally Benson gets by on very little sleep. In desperation, she once read a snowblower manual, hoping stupefaction would help her snooze.

According to the National Sleep Foundation, one in three American adults suffers at some time from insomnia, that catchall term for sleeplessness. Whatever the cause, insomnia looks like this: a delay of 30 minutes or more before falling asleep, frequent or prolonged awakening throughout the night, or early morning wake-ups.

Doctors don't consider insomnia chronic until it lasts about three weeks or more. But you should be concerned anytime poor sleep interferes with daytime functioning. According to the National Sleep Foundation, chronic insomniacs are more than twice as likely as sound sleepers to have a fatigue-related auto accident, and 25 percent less able to enjoy relationships with family and friends.

When Your Body Is Tired, but Your Mind Keeps Churning

Most insomniacs, say doctors, are driven sleepless by psychological rather than physical causes: for one-third to one-half, worry or depression is the culprit. For others, the cause may be pills or alcohol, or medical problems such as breathing ailments or chronic pain. Some people are just born poor sleepers, and in 10 percent of cases, body clocks veer off the normal cycle because of genetics or an odd schedule, such as working the graveyard shift.

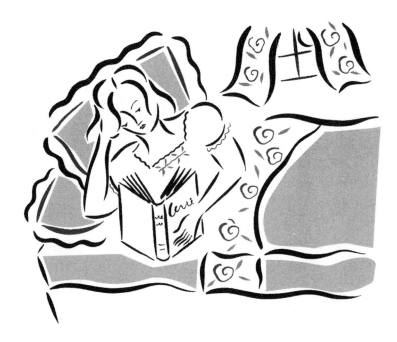

Although twice as many women as men report insomnia, it's not certain that they suffer from it more. Nor is it clear what role hormones play: While women often experience disturbed sleep during menopause and pregnancy and before their periods, researchers have yet to establish a link between hormonal fluctuations and insomnia. What is clear is that insomnia favors worriers, male or female. "Insomniacs say that if they could stop their thoughts, they could fall asleep," says William Finley, Ph.D., director of St. Mary's Sleep Disorders Center in Knoxville, Tennessee.

Insomnia often begins innocently: After a late dinner, we lie in bed, too full to sleep. What seemed so tasty an hour ago now stokes our metabolic furnace, triggering an increase in body temperature instead of the drop that sleep seeks. Gas or indigestion may add to our discomfort. So we lie awake obsessing about work, family or money. Near dawn we panic, sure no other human on earth is awake. Tomorrow is doomed; we'll feel lousy, look like a raccoon and perform like a sloth. Our body tunes in to our growing despair, our muscles tighten and our heart rate and body temperature climb—all of which ensures that sleep will remain out of reach.

For most, such nights are occasional and often linked to a specific anxiety—a new job, an unfamiliar bedroom. But for 10 to 15 percent of the population, the problem is chronic, outlasting the initial event by weeks, months or a lifetime.

How a person responds to occasional insomnia can influence whether the sleeplessness turns chronic. "Some people can adjust. They know the insomnia is temporary," says Charles Morin, Ph.D., professor of psychology at Laval University in Quebec City. "But other people begin worrying about whether they'll ever sleep well again. Or they think that because their spouse sleeps like a log, they should be able to."

These mistaken beliefs can act like mental neon signs, blinking us awake. In the last decade Dr. Morin and his colleagues have concentrated on reshaping misconceptions about sleep. Despite what you may have thought, for example, not all adults need eight hours to feel refreshed; some need only five or six, although doctors can't explain the variation.

INSIDE A SLEEP CLINIC

*C*arolyn Williams, 54, is smiling at the thought that she may actually sleep tonight. Since childhood, she's been up most nights, napping when she can—even at work. Five years ago sleeplessness finally forced her to quit her job, and she began coasting from doctor to doctor.

Now she's at St. Mary's in Knoxville, Tennessee, one of the 272 accredited sleep clinics nationwide. Of the 5 percent of people with sleep disorders who seek medical treatment, only a few—mostly those who suffer daytime sleepiness (narcolepsy) or whose spouses say they periodically stop breathing during sleep (sleep apnea)—end up at clinics. The cost: $30 to $130 for an initial evaluation, $1,700 and up for an overnight stay (during which technicians study brain waves, breathing patterns and muscle and eye movements).

Technicians attach electrodes to Williams's head for a computerized recording of her body signals. A camera aimed at the bed transmits to a control room where technicians will record Williams's every move.

Williams is on night two of a sleep study. The previous night, doctors discovered that she suffers from sleep apnea, so now a technician is fitting her for a mask connected to a blower that will drive air up her nose. Without the mask, called a CPAP, Williams's airway would collapse repeatedly during sleep. The near asphyxiation pumps adrenaline, making Williams wake up anxious.

Sleeping with a mask shooting air up your nose hardly sounds restful, but most patients adapt. And for Williams, the CPAP works. She sleeps through the night—for the first time she can remember in years. Elated, she packs her bag to leave. "I plan on having a normal life," she says, "whatever that is."

Rules to Snooze By

One of the most effective ways to beat insomnia is to practice what doctors call sleep hygiene. The basic rules:

Go to sleep and get up at the same time every day. Most of us push all week on six hours a night and sleep late on weekends. The result is a classic case of Sunday night insomnia. We hit the week building another bank of sleep debt that plays havoc with our body clocks. Regular sleeping hours prevent that.

Live life to the fullest. The more exciting your day, the deeper your sleep. "You can't watch TV all day and then sleep soundly," says Peter Hauri, Ph.D., director of the insomnia program at the Mayo Clinic in Rochester, Minnesota, and author of *No More Sleepless Nights*. Daily exercise should be part of that excitement, just not before bed. Working out five or six hours before sleep initially increases metabolism and body temperature, but lets them fall by bedtime.

Don't "work" at slumber. If you awaken, stay put for 15 minutes or so, says Dr. Finley. Chances are you'll fall back to sleep. But if you feel anxious or tense, get up and read until you feel sleepy again. Have a glass of milk if it helps, although the effect of nutrition on sleep remains anyone's guess. L-tryptophan, an amino acid in milk (as well as in beans and turkey), may make you drowsy, but there's not enough of the substance in one glass to help you doze. As a rule, don't go to bed hungry or stuffed.

Hide the clock. "Set the alarm and put it in the dresser across the room," says Dr. Hauri. "Whenever you look at the clock, you have an emotional reaction—worry that you haven't slept, happiness that you have—and emotion wakes you up."

It's also a good idea to check with a doctor for medical difficulties that could be causing insomnia (like a thyroid gone haywire) or psychological problems (like depression). If a doctor suspects a medical cause, she may refer you to a sleep center.

What *not* to do: self-medicate. Polishing off some wine may put you to sleep at first, but several hours later, as the alcohol withdraws from the brain, you'll pop awake. The sedating effects of over-the-counter sleeping pills can hang on for days. And while prescription pills may get us one good night's sleep, "when you stop taking them, you get rebound insomnia, a drug-withdrawal reaction," says Dr. Finley.

What the Experts Recommend

There are a number of doctor-recommended ways to battle insomnia.

Sleep-restriction therapy. This method helps reintroduce the insomniac to a good night's sleep and teaches her how much sleep she really needs. "If someone gets only six hours of sleep but spends nine hours in bed, my first instruction is to spend only six hours in bed," says Dr. Morin. Once the person is sleeping well for six hours, Dr. Morin adds 15 minutes each week until the patient sleeps soundly and wakes refreshed.

The Bootzin technique. This method tackles the conditioned anxiety many sleepless people develop about their beds. The trick is to reassociate the bed with comfort. Patients go to bed at the regular time but only if they're sleepy. If that "I can't sleep" panic starts, they leave the room. The next night they may sleep for five hours but then wake too early, feeling anxious. Again they leave the room. The process usually defangs the bedroom in two weeks to several months.

A daily dose of early morning sunlight. Doctors are not sure why it works, but they know sunlight interacts with the release of melatonin, a neurotransmitter that is released in the body when we're sleepy. Exposing someone to the light at 6:00 A.M. makes the melatonin release earlier, so the person feels sleepy earlier. (The daily dose of sunlight is about 80 to 100 times the intensity of indoor light.)

But whether what finally sends you to sleep is a boring novel, a cup of chamomile tea or a visit to a sleep clinic, you're bound to discover—and defeat—insomnia. Now, when Judith Evnen Benson wakes at night, she calms herself by saying, "It's the stay-awake bug telling me to get up." "Then I say, 'No, I'm not going to get into that,' and I roll over and go back to sleep." And most nights, she sleeps fine. "I just don't let myself wake up when I shouldn't," she says. And if she has to get up, she makes sure she doesn't take a step past 30.

PART THREE

Eating for Good Health

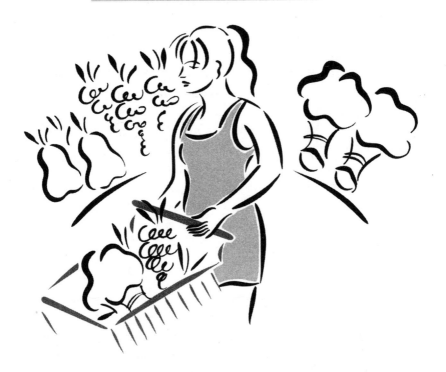

Foods That Help Turn Back the Clock

Want to live to a ripe old age? Load your shopping cart with this cornucopia of age-proofing produce.

Trying to get a handle on the foods that help you live longer can make you nuts. There you are in the produce aisle, searching your brain for a book's worth of information about which fruits and veggies are rich in bioflavonoids, which are booster shots of beta-carotene. Even with packaged food, many of the most important longevity nutrients don't show up on the labels.

Well, with the help of some of the nation's leading nutritionists, this royal pain becomes a no-brainer: Toss these 21 foods into your shopping cart every week, and you're covered—for all the vitamins, minerals, omega-3's and phytochemicals that have been shown to be long-life superstars.

Obviously, these aren't going to be the only foods you'll ever eat, and you don't have to eat each one every day. Simply follow the general longevity daily-diet guidelines of four or more fruits; six or more vegetables; eight or more servings of grains; ten or more helpings of nonmeat proteins (salmon, beans, tofu); plus a few doses of the little extras mentioned here (garlic, tea, flaxseed). Keep the menu varied so you work in some of everything each week, but don't get hung up on keeping track. After all, you don't need to be a nutritional bean counter for your diet to be among the healthiest and life-prolonging best.

Broccoli

Broccoli is the best one-stop vegetable munch for vitamins C and A, beta-carotene and fiber, according to nutritionist Melinda Morris, R.D., spokesperson for the Colorado Dietetic Association in Denver. Broccoli also contains a compound called sulforaphane, which has blocked the growth of breast tumors in mice. Great excuse to eat just the best parts: The highest levels of sulforaphane are in the florets, says Bronwyn G. Hughes, Ph.D., president of the Plant Bioactives Research Institute in Orem, Utah. Eat it raw for the most sulforaphane, but microwaving with a small amount of water retains up to 50 percent of it; boiling and steaming trail far behind, and commercially frozen broccoli has no detectable sulforaphane at all. *One serving = two or more spears*

Carrots

The equivalent of two carrots every second day provides enough beta-carotene to reduce stroke risk by half for men who have already had symptoms of heart disease, studies showed, and cut women's risk of stroke as well. *One serving = two medium carrots*

Chili Peppers

The heat source in chilies, capsaicin, is an antioxidant with a multitude of benefits: It protects DNA against carcinogens; it's a natural decongestant and expectorant; its blood-thinning ability helps prevent strokes; it lowers cholesterol. And some researchers believe capsaicin stimulates the release of the body's natural "feel good" chemicals, endorphins. *One serving = one or more peppers*

Spinach

One cup of raw spinach provides a bumper crop of vitamin A, vitamin C and folic acid, plus a bit of magnesium, which helps control cancer, reduces risk of stroke and heart disease, blocks free radicals and may help prevent osteoporosis. Dark green, leafy veg-

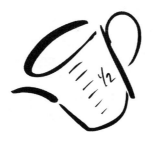

etables also contain glutathione, according to Patrick Quillin, R.D., Ph.D., vice-president of nutrition for The Cancer Treatment Centers of America. Glutathione helps make an enzyme that's important to immune system function. Fresh is best; cooking preserves little glutathione. *One serving = one cup, uncooked*

Mushrooms

"The basic mushroom that Americans find in their produce section may not be that valuable," Dr. Quillin says, but more exotic varieties contain beta-glucan, which acts like a vaccine to kick the immune system into higher gear. Shiitake, enoki, zhu ling and reishi, a type of hard, woody mushroom that grows on tree trunks, all have anti-cancer and antiviral effects. (*Note:* Never pick and eat wild mushrooms.) *One serving = ¼ cup dried shiitakes or three to six supplements*

Tomatoes or Strawberries

In a study of plants related to longevity, researchers found that the two that best correlated with a longer life were tomatoes and strawberries. Tomatoes are rich in lycopenes, an antioxidant even more potent than vitamin C that also stimulates immune system function and slows degenerative diseases. Tomatoes' only drawback is soft skin that may harbor fungicides, but soaking in water helps flush them out. Strawberries contain ellagic acid, which has been shown to have anti-cancer properties. *One serving = one fresh tomato or ½ cup strawberries*

Papaya, Pineapple or Kiwifruit

Enzymes, the catalysts that speed up the rate of reactions in the body, are found in high amounts in raw, fresh (and only raw, fresh) papaya, pineapple and kiwi, which help combat "everything from autoimmune diseases, allergies and cancer to AIDS," Dr. Quillin says. Three papayas a day would provide the dose that has shown dramatic effects against disease, but you can get the same benefit with kiwi and pineapple. *One serving = one papaya, one cup pineapple or one to two kiwis*

Mangoes

Although rich in carotenoids, mangoes don't have papaya's high enzyme levels. But they do contain another important category of phytochemical: bioflavonoids. Bioflavonoids help plants capture energy from the sun; when eaten, they aid our immune system and "they're antioxidants at least as effective as vitamin C and beta-carotene, if not more so," Dr. Quillin says. *One serving = one mango*

Citrus Fruits

Fresh, whole citrus fruits are a great source of vitamin C (oranges have the most), which more than 30 studies have shown helps the body fight cancers of the lung, cervix, esophagus and stomach. They're also extremely rich in bioflavonoids. The highest concentration is in the white rind, the part between the colored peel and the fruit, which means "when you drink orange juice, you're getting little or no bioflavonoids," Dr. Quillin says.

Limonene, a bioflavonoid found in the colored part of skin on citrus fruits, has been shown to be one of the most promising phytochemicals in the fight against cancer—it helped reverse cancer in animal studies. But don't eat the entire fruit, peel and all, because of sprayed-on pesticides. *One serving = one large orange or equivalent fruit*

Cantaloupe

One-quarter melon delivers 2 milligrams of beta-carotene—nearly half the National Cancer Institute's recommended 5.7 milligrams per day for cancer prevention and protection against heart disease. Cantaloupe is also a rich source of vitamin C. *One serving = ¼ melon*

Apricots

Fresh apricots are high in beta-carotene and provide medium-high levels of vitamin C and some fiber. Vitamin C vanishes from dried apricots, and if they're untreated, they lose beta-carotene as well. Nonorganic dried apricots (and other dried fruits) treated with sulphur dioxide retain their beta-carotene, but the chemical can cause asthma in some people, Dr. Quillin says. *One serving = three apricots*

Bananas

Bananas are rich in magnesium (shown to help protect the circulatory system), potassium and slowly absorbed simple sugars. They're also a good source of pectin, a soluble fiber that prevents radical swings in blood sugar. *One serving = one medium banana*

Garlic

"Garlic is a powerhouse of antioxidants of various kinds," says Jean Carper, syndicated food-nutrition columnist and author of *Food—Your Miracle Medicine*. "There have been lots of studies that show it lowers cholesterol, lowers blood pressure, is an antiviral and antibacterial, and it may have chemicals capable of destroying cancer cells, even after you get cancer."

Dr. Quillin offers a good way to eat garlic: Place unpeeled garlic cloves in a microwave-safe cup, sprinkle with olive oil, cover loosely with plastic wrap and microwave for about 30 seconds. Slip the peel off and eat a few with meals—"it tastes somewhat like cashews." A bonus: less offensive garlic breath. *One serving = two to three cloves of fresh garlic, one teaspoon of garlic powder, four one-gram powdered*

garlic tablets, four gel caps of Kyolic garlic or one teaspoon of liquid Kyolic garlic

Tea

Drinking five cups of tea is equal to eating two vegetables, or nearly half of the minimum daily intake recommended by the latest nutrition guidelines, according to John Weisburger, M.D., Ph.D., senior member of the American Health Foundation in Valhalla, New York. Tea is loaded with antioxidants called polyphenols, and "there is some evidence from numerous laboratory studies that both green tea and black tea reduce heart disease, cancer and stroke risk, and it even shows some promise as an antagonist against certain viruses," he says. Green and black tea both have "roughly the same effect" (and it doesn't matter how you drink it). *One serving = one cup*

Beans

Nutritionist Morris says that although there is no single most important food, if she were forced to select one, it'd be beans. They're high in protein and complex carbohydrates, have both soluble and insoluble fiber and are filling, cheap and taste good. Beans are loaded with phytochemicals and protease inhibitors that may help prevent cancer, says Phyllis E. Bowen, Ph.D., associate professor of human nutrition and dietetics at the University of Illinois at Chicago.

If you don't like beans, try pasta made from lupine beans. It's rich in fiber, carotenes and high-quality proteins and contains twice the calcium of other nondairy foods, according to researchers at North Dakota State University in Fargo. *One serving = one cup*

Soybeans and Tofu

Tofu, fresh soybeans, soy milk and soy protein isolates (a commercial product that's 90 percent protein) decrease "bad" low-density lipoprotein (LDL) cholesterol levels in blood, which reduces heart disease risk. Even moderate amounts help, but the more people eat, the more dramatically their cholesterol drops, according to a study by Sue Potter, Ph.D., assistant professor of food and nutrition at the University of Illinois at Urbana-Champaign. Soy is also high in phytoestrogens, a category of bioflavonoids that inhibit estrogen-promoted cancers and protect against radiation in chemotherapy. Studies have shown that regular soy-eaters have reduced risk or lower rates of prostate, colon, lung, rectal and stomach cancers. *One serving = up to four ounces of tofu or equivalent soy product*

Salmon

In addition to salmon's well-known heart-disease-fighting omega-3 oils, it has calcium, magnesium, complete proteins and B vitamins. Its B_6 serves as another buffer against heart disease, boosts the immune system, stimulates an enzyme that regulates the nervous system and helps to prevent some cancers. Salmon even has carotenoids, which account for its orange-pink color, notes dietitian Susan Adams, R.D., a nutritional sciences lecturer at the University of Washington in Seattle. *One serving = three ounces*

Flaxseed

Flaxseed is very high in oil, says Dr. Bowen—but that's good: 51 percent of the oil is linolenic acid, "so if you can't eat fish, that's the way to get your omega-3 oils." Like soybeans, flaxseed also has phytoestrogens called lignans, which have been linked to breast and colon cancer prevention, Dr. Bowen adds.

One good way to get your flaxseed is through whole-grain breads made with flaxseed meal; check labels. *One serving = two tablespoons*

Oats

Researchers have found that oat bran lowers cholesterol and blood pressure and may also be beneficial in reducing the chances of colon cancer. Oatmeal contains both soluble and insoluble fiber, but it's the soluble fiber in oatmeal that provides the most health benefits. *One serving = one cup oats or oatmeal; 1½ packets of instant oatmeal or 1¼ cups oat flakes cereal*

Quinoa

A staple that nourished the ancient Incas, quinoa (pronounced KEEN-wa) is one of the best plant protein sources, featuring a complete selection of amino acids, high calcium, fiber, phosphorus, iron and lysine. Quinoa can be cooked like rice (only faster) or bought as a flour for baking. "A lot of people don't know how to cook quinoa," says Michele Lubin, research nutritionist at the American Health Foundation, "but it's really easy to make." *One serving = ½ to one cup*

Wheat Germ

With 24 grams of protein per half-cup, wheat germ is a great addition to the grains tier of our dietary pyramid. It's also a good source of disease-fighting nutrients such as B vitamins, calcium and magnesium. But it's the oil in wheat germ that makes it the richest food source for vitamin E, which enhances immune function and, as an antioxidant, helps prevent cataracts and atherosclerosis. *One serving = ½ cup*

Nutrients That Youthify Your Body

Research suggests that antioxidants like vitamins A, C and E act like nature's preservatives, slowing or reversing aging.

*I*f you're in search of the Fountain of Youth, look no farther than your nearest supermarket. Because, believe it or not, what you put in your cart—and, later, in your mouth—can affect how long and healthy your life will be.

Scientists now believe that the vitamins and minerals in foods play a role in the health and vigor of every part of the body, including your skin, heart, bones and brain. What's more, eating the right foods can protect you from many illnesses, such as heart disease, cancer, arthritis, osteoporosis and cataracts. And consuming healthful foods can also speed wound healing, fortify your immune system and keep your teeth and gums in top condition.

"In many cases, nutrition is a new form of medicine," says William Pryor, Ph.D., professor of chemistry and biochemistry and director of the Biodynamics Institute at Louisiana State University in Baton Rouge. "We're finding that the effects of certain nutrients are quite potent and, in many cases, will reduce the incidence of disease by about 50 percent."

So because a healthful diet decreases your chances of developing illnesses, chances are you'll live longer. But there's more good news: Some doctors believe that healthful eating may also slow the general decline of body functions which we refer to as the aging process.

What's the bottom line for people who want to modify their diet to put the brakes on aging and disease? Make sure you're consuming enough of the vitamins and minerals that can keep your body strong. Here's a rundown of some of the most important nutrients, how they work to keep your body young and which foods contain them.

Beta-Carotene: Cellular "Cement"

Some of the most potent time-defying nutrients are the antioxidants, such as beta-carotene. The body converts this antioxidant into a form of vitamin A. Beta-carotene protects the body's tissues from degeneration, boosts the immune system, protects against cancer, heart disease and stroke, maintains good vision and keeps skin healthy.

Good sources of beta-carotene include apricots and peaches, cantaloupe, carrots, dark green vegetables, such as kale, spinach and broccoli, pumpkin and winter squash and sweet potatoes.

Vitamin E: The Heart Helper

This antioxidant has a great reputation for foiling free radicals, chemicals that occur naturally in your body and can lead to the death of healthy body cells. Vitamin E soaks up free radicals, protecting cells from damage and possibly extending the cells' life spans.

Vitamin E also reduces the risk of coronary heart disease and angina, which is a severe pain in the heart muscle that occurs when the heart doesn't receive enough oxygen. (One theory is that vitamin

A RADICAL SOLUTION

Antioxidants—including beta-carotene, selenium, zinc and vitamins E and C—are some of the most important anti-aging nutrients. Here's why: When your body performs normal processes such as metabolism and detoxification (breaking down toxic chemicals), your cells give off by-products called free radicals. These by-products are highly reactive agents that can cause chemical chain reactions that ultimately lead to the death of healthy body cells. While the demise of a few cells won't be lethal to the person who's losing them, damage will accumulate over the years. And some scientists believe that it's this accumulation of cell death that may be the cause of many of the degenerative processes that we call aging.

Enter the antioxidants to save the day—and your youth. These dietary heroes are nutrients that help slow down or prevent the free radicals from wreaking their havoc on your healthy cells. The antioxidants bond with the free radicals, which renders them harmless and stops the damaging chain reaction before it begins.

Each antioxidant seems to work in a different way to counteract free-radical damage. So they're all important, explains Jeffrey Blumberg, Ph.D., associate director of the United States Department of Agriculture's Human Nutrition Research Center on Aging at Tufts University in Boston. Some of the specific benefits your body reaps from antioxidants are a reduced risk of atherosclerosis (the underlying cause of heart disease), a strengthened immune system and a decreased risk of macular degeneration (an age-related disease that causes eyesight to deteriorate).

E helps keep blood from clotting too easily, which allows it to flow through narrowed coronary arteries.) In addition, E boosts the immune system and protects against cataracts and cancer.

Foods rich in E include dark green, leafy vegetables, nuts such as almonds, filberts, peanuts and pecans, shrimp, sweet potatoes, vegetable oils, wheat germ and whole grains.

Vitamin C: The Great Protector

Research suggests that this antioxidant boosts high-density lipoprotein (HDL) cholesterol (the "good" cholesterol that prevents clogged arteries) and puts the brakes on low-density lipoprotein (LDL) cholesterol (the kind that creates the artery blockages that lead to heart attack and stroke). What's more, vitamin C boosts the immune system, guards against cancer, keeps gums and teeth healthy, prevents cataracts, speeds wound healing, counteracts asthma and prevents infertility in men by maintaining sperm quality.

Foods rich in vitamin C include broccoli, cauliflower, citrus fruits and juices, cantaloupe, honeydew and watermelon, red and green peppers, strawberries and tomatoes.

Selenium: The Immunity Booster

Selenium works its anti-aging magic in a more roundabout way than its sister antioxidants. It helps produce a special enzyme, which, in turn, transforms certain free radicals into harmless water. The result is a fortified immune system, a decreased risk of heart disease and stroke, and protection from cancers of the colon, rectum and lungs.

To be sure you're consuming enough selenium, include the following in your diet: broccoli, celery, cucumbers, fish, lobster and shrimp, mushrooms and whole-grain cereals and breads.

Zinc: For People on the Mend

Not only is zinc a part of an enzyme that protects cells against free radicals, but it's also capable of working as an antioxidant itself. Your body relies on a steady supply of this mineral to keep your immune system healthy. What's more, zinc helps to heal wounds by aiding in the manufacture of new cells.

Keep zinc in your diet by eating extra-lean beef, liver and poultry, fish and oysters, legumes and nuts, low-fat or nonfat cheese and whole-grain breads.

Vitamin B$_6$: An Aid to Sharp-Thinking

This vitamin may help keep your mind sharp and strengthen your immune system. A word of caution, however: Vitamin B6 can be toxic in high doses. Consult your doctor before taking supplements of this vitamin.

To get enough B$_6$ through diet alone, try bananas and plantains,

THE FORGOTTEN NUTRIENT

*W*hen you're gobbling up the healthful foods listed in this chapter, don't forget to wash them down with a big glass of water. On average, we lose two to three quarts every day—and most folks don't drink enough to replace what they lose. "The average person is a pint short on water each day, which puts stress on the kidneys," says George Blackburn, M.D., Ph.D., chief of the nutrition/metabolism laboratory at Deaconess Hospital in Boston. Caffeine-containing beverages such as coffee, tea and some sodas don't help: They're diuretics, which speed up water loss. To maintain a healthy fluid intake, wet your whistle with water whenever possible. Or down a big glass of H_2O before you start sipping on something else.

chicken, fish and lean pork, oats and whole-wheat products, peanuts, walnuts and soybeans and whole-grain rice.

Vitamin B_{12}: Nature's Battery Charger

This B vitamin may help keep your mind sharp and your energy reserves high. While your body needs very little of this vitamin, alcohol and certain medications can hinder its absorption.

To be sure you're getting all the B_{12} you need, include the following in your diet: eggs, extra-lean beef and liver, fish and low-fat and nonfat dairy products. (If you have reason to lower your intake of dietary cholesterol, keep your consumption of eggs to a minimum.)

Calcium: A Woman's Health Protector

This mineral makes for strong bones, but it also helps boost muscle power and nerve function. Getting adequate calcium is essential for everyone. It's particularly crucial for women, however, because they're at higher risk of losing bone tissue and developing the brittle-bone condition known as osteoporosis.

In addition, calcium may help alleviate premenstrual symptoms, including irritability, anxiousness and depression, as well as cramps, backaches and headaches. And eating calcium-rich foods may help lower mild high blood pressure to normal levels. Foods rich in calcium include broccoli, leafy greens such as collards and kale, legumes such as pinto beans and lentils, low-fat and nonfat dairy products and tofu made with calcium carbonate.

Iron: Critical for Stamina

The mineral iron operates in virtually every part of the body, providing it with the oxygen needed for metabolism. Women, who require more of this mineral than men do, often don't consume enough iron. This leaves them at risk for anemia—a condition characterized by feelings of extreme fatigue, headaches and body chills.

To keep your body healthy and stave off anemia, be sure to include the following in your diet: breads, dark-meat poultry, extra-lean meats, fish, iron-fortified cereals and legumes.

Including the above nutrients in your daily diet will go a long way toward keeping your body healthy and youthful for years to come. Bon appétit!

The World's Healthiest Diet?

Japanese women are less likely to develop breast and other forms of cancer than American women—and they live longer, too.

The Japanese are known for many things: electronics, cars, making a multimillion-dollar deal with Michael Jackson. But their most amazing accomplishment is living long, healthy lives. Japanese women live an average of 82½ years; men, 76 years. By comparison, American women live 79 years; American men, 72. More important, Japanese mortality rates for many cancers are among the lowest in the industrial world. For example, the Japanese death rate from breast cancer is about one-fourth of ours (6.3 women per 100,000, compared with 22.4 here).

So why hasn't someone figured out what makes them live so long and made a pill out of it? Because it's difficult when confronted with broad epidemiological evidence—that is, the basic data that describe large populations—for scientists to tease out exactly what is causing the differences between groups. The most likely candidate is usually arrived at by a process of elimination.

If longevity were bestowed by genetics, for example, you would expect the Japanese to live longer even if they left their homeland. But when Japanese men migrate to the United States, their death rate from prostate cancer converges with that of American-born men. The same is true of Japanese women and breast cancer.

The environment probably isn't responsible for these differences either. Japan has its share of pollutants and carcinogens. Nor is the modern Japanese lifestyle any less stressful than that of the West. That leaves diet.

A Centuries-Old Diet

Most nutrition experts believe that the Japanese are healthier and live longer because of what they eat. Their traditional diet differs

CANCER RATES IN WOMEN:
UNITED STATES VERSUS JAPAN

The American Cancer Society surveyed 46 countries from 1988 to 1991 to find out where people were most likely to die of various cancers. The lower the number, the higher the incidence of cancer. Here are the figures for women in the United States and Japan.

Cancer	United States	Japan
All types	11th	44th
Colon	19th	32nd
Lung	2nd	23rd
Breast	16th	44th
Uterine	33rd	37th
Stomach	46th	5th
Leukemia	9th	44th

greatly from Western diets, and when the Japanese abandon it, their health suffers.

Breakfast is a bowl of rice, a small piece of fish and a bowl of dashi—a soup based on fish stock and miso with a little seaweed floating in it.

Lunch may be a bowl of noodles in broth garnished with vegetables or tofu. Or it could be a small meal brought to work as a *bento* (a box lunch) that may contain rice balls wrapped in seaweed, a little fish and some leftovers.

An ordinary home-cooked dinner is yet another bowl of rice, miso soup and a few side dishes—pickled vegetables, fish, seaweed, tofu, perhaps a little meat—followed by green tea and fruit.

This is the diet most people in Japan have been eating for hundreds—perhaps thousands—of years. Meat is always used in small quantities, prepared and eaten lean. Dairy products are still relatively rare. Refined sugar is used sparingly. Fried foods and breads and other baked goods play a minor role in a cuisine that relies on a wide variety of cooking methods. The Japanese consume a lot of soy. And green tea—not soda—is the national beverage.

Add Fish, Subtract Salt

It should come as no surprise that diet could be central to good health. Every year, new studies remind us that fat consumption promotes heart disease and perhaps certain types of cancer, and that consuming too much refined sugar over time may set the stage for diabetes. There is evidence that phytochemicals—beta-carotene is one—in fruits and vegetables may inhibit cancers. And we're only beginning to understand the possible impact of omega-3 fatty acids on health.

But these same studies also make it increasingly clear that there is no nutritional magic bullet: Good health is the result of total diet and lifestyle. A low-fat, high-fiber diet—with lots of vegetables and very little meat—as part of a tobacco-free, active life can improve the odds that you will live longer and, even better, be healthier over the entire span of your life. That's why Japanese cuisine makes such an appealing model: Although it includes small amounts of meat, it could easily be adapted to the perfect, meatless diet.

To get to that perfect diet, you'd have to make only a few changes. The Japanese diet includes few fresh fruits and vegetables, in part because the islands lack the agricultural land to grow them. The Japanese preserve all sorts of foods by pickling them, a process that often relies on salt. In fact, scientists blame consumption of salt for Japan's traditionally high rates of stroke, hypertension and stomach cancer. And as the Japanese have become more affluent, they have begun eating more animal protein and fat—with devastating results. Heart disease, once virtually unheard of in Japan, is now a major concern; breast cancer mortality rates almost doubled between 1935 and 1980.

Still, we would do well to emulate much of Japan's traditional diet. All of the following foods, which are staples of the cuisine, are loaded with potential health benefits and have yielded such promising results in laboratory research that each component, at one time or another, has been given credit for keeping Japanese cancer and heart disease rates down.

Amazing Soy

The United States grows half the soybeans in the world, about 50 million metric tons. Most of these are fed to animals. The rest are exported to countries like Japan, where people consume them in many forms—as flour, oil, sauce, tofu—to their great benefit.

Soy foods are lavishly endowed with the hottest potential anticarcinogen since beta-carotene—an isoflavone called genistein. It is one of soy's five phytochemicals. These plant chemicals naturally protect the plant against disease and may enhance human immunity when we consume them. In more than 30 studies, genistein has been shown to inhibit the growth of cancer cells in the lab. German researchers found that people who ate a traditional Japanese diet had at least 30 times the amount of genistein in their urine as Westerners did and discovered that the substance blocks the growth of new blood vessels, which is necessary for the development of many kinds of tumors. So far, soy is the only food in which genistein has been found in high concentrations.

Another way genistein and other isoflavones may protect health is through their ability to block the effect of estrogen. In animal and laboratory studies, isoflavones have been shown to bind to estrogen receptors on certain cells, preventing the buildup of natural estrogens that may play a role in some cancers.

While there is as yet no conclusive proof that genistein and other phytochemicals retard cancer, the link between soy and lower cholesterol rates is easier to prove. "Studies show a 15 percent decrease in cholesterol levels when soy is added to the diet," says Mark Messina, Ph.D., author of *The Simple Soybean and Your Health*. But it takes quite a bit of soy—20 to 25 grams a day, or the equivalent of two to three servings of tofu—to bring cholesterol levels down.

It may take only four ounces of tofu or eight ounces of soybean milk a day to reduce cancer risk. Other ways to incorporate soy are by using soy oil in salad dressings and soy flour in recipes. But increasing consumption of soy should be just one part of a better eating plan. Dr. Messina notes: "It's not enough to wash down your Big Mac and fries with a glass of soybean milk."

More Disease-Fighting Foods

Soy is not the only health-promoting component of the Japanese diet. There's some evidence that the following foods can help protect your health as well.

Rice and noodles. These complex carbohydrates, high in fiber and a variety of nutrients, form the centerpiece of the Japanese diet. Among fiber's many benefits: It dilutes the concentration of carcinogenic compounds in the colon, moves everything through the system faster, maintains a healthy balance between harmful and benign bacteria in the digestive system and may help to lower cholesterol levels.

Polished white rice is by far the most important food in Japan. (The Japanese avoid brown rice because they associate it with poverty. However, it is a superior source of vitamins, minerals and protein, and has two to three times the fiber of white rice.) While rice doesn't have a lot of protein, what it has is of very high quality—meaning it contains near-optimal proportions of most of the essential amino acids that your body needs. "Rice and soy work beautifully together to form a complete protein," says Paul A. LaChance, Ph.D., chair of the department of food science at Rutgers University in New Brunswick, New Jersey.

Japanese noodles are made without eggs, and are usually served in broth or accompanied by a dipping sauce, both of which are typically low in fat. Although thick *udon* and *somen* noodles, both made with white wheat flour, are the most popular varieties in Japan, *soba* noodles are nutritionally superior. Thin, brownish soba noodles, made of wheat or buckwheat, have an almost perfect amino acid balance. They are rich in vitamin C and riboflavin, low in fat and sodium.

Fish. "There's much more fish eaten regularly in Japan than in any other country in the world, except maybe Portugal and Iceland," says nutritional epidemiologist Lawrence Kushi, Sc.D., of the University of Minnesota in Minneapolis. Because fish is relatively low in fat and high in omega-3 fatty acids, it may play a role in the traditionally low heart disease and overall cancer rates in Japan.

Dried fish, one of the basic ingredients in stocks and soups, is not as healthful, however. And eating raw fish can be a bit risky—larval-stage parasitic worms may lurk in sushi and sashimi, but at worst they cause abdominal pain. The parasites are killed when the raw fish is frozen (at -4°F for seven days in home freezers), and the freezing, if done properly, doesn't affect the flavor of the fish.

Green tea. Japan's national beverage is sipped moderately hot, without sugar or milk. Numerous animal studies have shown it to be protective against cancers of the skin, colon, breast, lung, esophagus and liver. Epidemiological studies corroborate these results. "The polyphenols in tea are powerful antioxidants," says John H. Weisburger, M.D., Ph.D., senior member of the American Health Foundation in Valhalla, New York. Black tea appears to do the job just as well as green: "The polyphenols in black tea have a chemical structure that is just as active in disease prevention," says Dr. Weisburger. And they remain intact in the decaffeination process. Because tea is a plant extract, Weisburger claims, anyone who uses five tea bags a day—black, green or decaffeinated—is getting a benefit equivalent to eating two servings of fruits or vegetables.

Seaweed or sea vegetables. Neither true weeds nor true vegetables, sea vegetables are algae. Virtually everyone in Japan eats them daily. Some Japanese researchers claim sea vegetables contain more minerals than any other kind of food, among them calcium, magnesium, sodium, potassium, iodine, iron, zinc, copper and selenium. Calcium and iron, which Westerners tend to get from animal protein, are particularly abundant in most sea vegetables.

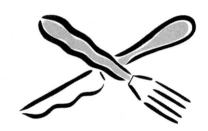

Studies have found sea vegetables effective in reducing cholesterol and in helping to prevent hypertension and atherosclerosis. There is also evidence that seaweed might protect against colon, prostate and breast cancers. Researchers have found that kombu, or kelp, delays and reduces breast tumors in rats. Scientists speculate that sea vegetables boost immunity, have antibiotic properties and diminish the impact environmental pollutants have on health.

Take a Hint from Japan

Obviously, the Japanese diet emphasizes foods, such as seaweed and soy, that we eat rarely or not at all. And it virtually excludes major features of our daily fare, such as dairy products, refined sugar and large quantities of animal protein.

But it's not just the specific foods that make Japan's traditional diet superior to ours, although there are no better sources of the nutrients that encourage good health than soy, rice and sea vegetables. It's the way they view food, too: small portions, artistic presentation, a great variety of ingredients. In other words, you don't have to frequent a sushi bar to reap the benefits of the Japanese diet. Try keeping your foods low in fat and animal protein, emphasize balance and diversity, avoid overeating and, perhaps most important, enjoy your meal.

Eat to Energize!

Do you lose steam by mid-morning? Poop out after lunch? Changing your diet may help you boost energy that's gone bust.

If you blame your lack of energy on your busy schedule and assume you were born this way, think again. Fatigue is not normal, and you don't have to take it lying down. Often a few simple changes in what or how you eat is all it takes to put the spring back into your step.

The Fastest Way to Energize

There are hundreds of excuses for not eating breakfast, but none of them is worth the cost to your energy level and general well-being. Breakfast is just that: It breaks the overnight fast and restocks your dwindling energy stores.

Skipping breakfast because you're not hungry could be a conditioned response. "Your stomach knocks on the appetite door as if to say 'I'm hungry,' but if no one is listening, the hunger pangs eventually go away," says nutritionist Evelyn Tribole, R.D., a dietitian in Beverly Hills, California, and author of *Intuitive Eating* and nutritionist for "Good Morning America." In short, your body needs the fuel, but you're ignoring the signals.

Ironically, people who skip breakfast in an effort to cut calories often do more snacking later in the day and overeat at evening meals. Breakfast is one way to evenly distribute your day's calories and nutrients and help maintain a steady blood sugar and energy level.

The first step in feeling better is to eat breakfast, even if you're not hungry. The three rules for planning breakfast are:

1. Make it light.
2. Limit the fat.
3. Include a protein-rich food and a carbohydrate-rich food.

The balance of carbohydrates and protein is critical. If you eat too little protein, you're likely to feel hungry within a few hours, while too much carbohydrate is likely to make you sleepy by midmorning. Meals with a mix of protein and starch maintain blood sugar and energy levels for up to four hours or more.

Also, avoid high-sugar breakfasts such as doughnuts and coffee, which trigger an initial energy boost but leave you drowsy within a few hours.

Caution: Coffee Can Leave You Logey

Coffee's welcoming aroma and promise of instant energy have made it the number one mind-altering drug and the second most popular beverage, just behind soft drinks, in the United States. Americans consume 450 cups of coffee per person per year.

FATIGUE-FIGHTING BREAKFASTS YOU'LL *WANT* TO EAT

*H*ere are some quick and easy low-fat breakfast ideas that offer a combination of protein and carbohydrates.

- Fill a crepe with low-fat ricotta cheese and fruit.
- Fill a tortilla with shredded carrots, zucchini, low-fat cheese and salsa.
- Have a cup of vegetable soup with cheese and bread.
- Mix fresh fruit into vanilla yogurt.

- Top an English muffin with one ounce of nonfat cheese and broil until bubbly. Serve with a glass of orange juice.
- Toast a frozen whole-wheat waffle and top it with fat free sour cream and fresh blueberries.
- Warm a low-fat bran muffin and serve with applesauce and yogurt.

Coffee isn't all bad. Some people report that they think faster, work more efficiently, concentrate better and are more alert after drinking one or two cups. But when intake creeps above moderate, the initial high is followed by mild withdrawal symptoms, one of which is fatigue. A vicious cycle can result as a person drinks more coffee to prevent the inevitable letdown.

Caffeine also lingers in the body for three to four hours. As a consequence, coffee drinkers take longer to fall asleep, sleep less soundly, wake up more often and wake up groggier than nondrinkers. Substituting a cup of tea or a diet cola for an evening cup of coffee will not prevent insomnia, however, since both contain the same amount of caffeine as a cup of instant coffee.

By the way, caffeine is also found in cocoa, coffee-flavored ice cream and yogurt, chocolate and many over-the-counter medications, including headache remedies.

Advice for Java Junkies

There's no need to give up coffee—just cut back. One to three five-ounce cups, or the equivalent of 300 milligrams of caffeine or less, in the morning or early afternoon appear to be safe and, except for the most sensitive people, should not contribute to fatigue.

Because coffee is a diuretic, it can contribute to dehydration and, subsequently, fatigue. Be sure to drink additional water and other fluids during the day to make up for fluids lost from drinking coffee.

People struggling with fatigue who drink a lot of coffee should gradually reduce their intake by one or two cups a day. They are most likely to feel tired or experience other symptoms of coffee withdrawal, such as headaches, if coffee intake is reduced too quickly.

Another suggestion for reducing but not eliminating coffee is to switch to instant coffee or an instant coffee blended with chicory or grain. These coffees contain half the caffeine of regular brews. Or blend regular and decaffeinated coffee before brewing, or have your coffee shop combine regular and decaf.

Sweets Can Slow You Down

Do you grab a candy bar when you feel tired? Do you soothe your weary mind with a doughnut? These quick fixes offer a temporary high that could actually be fueling your fatigue.

Researchers at Kansas State University measured mood in 120 women who drank 12 ounces of water or beverages sweetened with either aspartame (NutraSweet) or sugar. Within 30 minutes the women who drank the sugar-sweetened drink were the drowsiest.

Why do sweets bring you down? For one thing, unlike starch, which slowly releases carbohydrate units called glucose into the blood, sugar dumps rapidly into the bloodstream, causing a rapid rise in blood sugar. To counteract this rise, the pancreas quickly releases insulin, which shuttles excess sugar from the blood into the cells. Consequently, blood sugar drops, often to levels lower than before the snack.

Sugar also increases tryptophan levels in the brain and triggers the release of the brain chemical serotonin, which in turn slows you down. Harris R. Lieberman, Ph.D., a research scientist, and Bonnie Spring, Ph.D., professor of psychology, both at the Massachusetts Institute of Technology in Cambridge, report that people feel sleepier and have "less vigor" for up to 3½ hours after eating a highly refined carbohydrate snack, as compared to one that contains more protein.

ARE YOU SUGAR-SENSITIVE?

*E*very condition from fatigue to personality disorders has been blamed on hypoglycemia, or low blood sugar. Hypoglycemia is not a disease but a symptom of abnormal blood sugar regulation. It is common in diabetics and people with some other conditions. Documented symptoms of hypoglycemia include fatigue, irritability, inability to concentrate, headaches, palpitations, perspiration, anxiety, hunger and shakiness. Many more people believe they have hypoglycemia, however, than actually test positive when given a blood sugar test.

The best dietary advice for sugar-sensitive people is to consume five or six small meals throughout the day, rather than a few large meals. In addition, they should consume some complex carbohydrate, protein and fiber at each meal and snack. The soluble fibers found in oranges, apples, legumes and oats are particularly effective in slowing the absorption of sugar and allow a slow, steady release of sugar into the blood.

Finally, people who frequently snack on sweets are likely to consume inadequate amounts of the energizing nutrients. Researchers at the Division of Human Nutrition in Adelaide, Australia, report that the more sugar people consume, the higher their fat and calorie consumption and the lower their intake of vitamins and minerals—in particular, vitamin C, beta-carotene, the B vitamins, magnesium, potassium and zinc.

In the long run, consuming sugar as a quick fix for dwindling energy can initiate a vicious cycle. "The person suffering from chronic tiredness and depression who turns to sugary foods may relieve the fatigue and feel better for a short while, but the depression and fatigue return," says Larry Christensen, Ph.D., chair of the Department of Psychology at the University of South Alabama in Mobile. The person then must either reach for another sugar fix or seek help elsewhere.

Eliminating sugar and caffeine from the diet is a permanent solution. Or simply snack defensively rather than feeding your fatigue.

STAY-ALERT SNACKS

*W*ant an energizing snack? Try the following:

- Fruit juice or fresh fruit, peanut butter and crackers
- Whole-wheat bread sticks and nonfat cheese
- English muffin with all-fruit jam and fat-free cream cheese
- Fruit-filled crepe
- Miniature raisin bagel with fat-free cream cheese
- Soft microwave pretzel
- Hot or cold baked potato with nonfat sour cream or nonfat cottage cheese
- Pita bread stuffed with shredded jalapeno cheese and zucchini
- Flavored rice cakes dipped in yogurt
- Baby carrots

Lunch: Eat Light and Stay Awake

Even if you eat a nutritious breakfast and snack in the morning, your energy could diminish as the day progresses if you don't stop to refuel. What and how you eat for lunch could determine how you feel by midafternoon.

Keep lunch light. A low-fat midday meal that contains approximately 500 calories maintains afternoon alertness and boosts energy levels, while skipping lunch or indulging in a high-fat, high-calorie lunch of 1,000 calories or more can leave you yawning.

Carbohydrate-rich foods also can elevate serotonin levels and make you drowsy, while protein-rich foods increase the brain level of the amino acid tyrosine, a primary building block for the energizing chemicals dopamine and norepinephrine. In studies, tyrosine was found to boost alertness, vigilance and concentration.

Consequently, plan your carbohydrates so they work with your energy levels, not against them. For example, you may feel relaxed after a carbohydrate-rich dinner of spaghetti, but the same meal at lunch could make you sluggish. Light lunches, such as a tuna sandwich with fruit and low-fat milk, or a salad with French bread and yogurt, are more likely to keep you going throughout the afternoon. Other "brain power" foods include a small amount of fish, skinless chicken, or legumes combined with grains and vegetables.

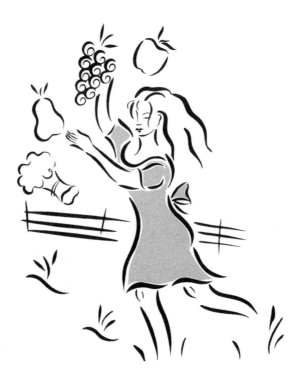

People who crave carbohydrates are an exception to the rule. According to researchers at the Massachusetts Institute of Technology in Cambridge, people who crave sweet or starchy foods in the afternoon might have extra-low levels of serotonin. While others feel drowsy, carbohydrate cravers are energized and more alert after they eat carbohydrates, especially if they are complex carbohydrates such as cereals, breads, pasta or starchy vegetables.

If you crave carbohydrates, don't expect to "will away" those cravings. Make sure every lunch contains some complex carbohydrates, such as a baked potato topped with grated vegetables and low-fat cheese. And plan to include a carbohydrate-rich snack for your midday doldrums. You might eat 20 to 30 flavored miniature rice cakes, a handful of pretzels, a banana or a bagel.

Top Ten Tips for an Energizing Lifestyle

Whether you're an early bird or a night owl, the following rules can help boost your energy level.

YOU SNOOZE, YOU LOSE—ENERGY, THAT IS

*T*he link is clear: People who exercise feel more energetic, while the sedentary get drowsier. Exercise increases blood flow to the muscles and brain, releases energizing hormones and stimulates the nervous system to produce chemicals, called endorphins, that elevate mood and produce feelings of well-being.

In one study, 18 people rated their energy levels after 12 days of either eating a candy bar or walking briskly for ten minutes. Results indicated that walking increases energy levels and lowers tension, while a sugary snack increases feelings of tension and only temporarily raises energy levels, followed by an increase in fatigue and reduced energy. So when you feel like lying down, try getting up and moving around instead.

1. At breakfast, eat at least one serving of protein-rich foods such as legumes, meats or low-fat dairy and at least two servings of fruits, vegetables and grains.
2. Limit caffeinated beverages to three servings or fewer and don't drink tea and coffee with meals.
3. Never eat sugar alone and limit your daily intake to 10 percent of total calories.
4. Eat several small meals and snacks approximately every four hours.
5. Eat a moderate-size, low-fat lunch that contains a mixture of protein and carbohydrates.
6. If you crave carbohydrates, plan a carbohydrate-rich snack for your low-energy period of the day.
7. Do not overeat in the evening and avoid excessive snacking after dinner.
8. Avoid severe calorie-restricted diets. People who repeatedly diet or consume very low calorie diets report that they have trouble concentrating, experience impaired judgment and have poor memory.
9. Drink at least six to eight glasses of water a day. Chronic low fluid intake is a common but often overlooked cause of mild dehydration and fatigue.

10. Limit your alcohol consumption. Alcohol dehydrates the cells and suppresses the nervous system, causing poor attention, fatigue and sleep disturbances.

Which Vitamins Do You Need?

Sure, swallowing a supplement every day is simpler than eating right. But is it a substitute for real food?

Vitamin supplements are big business these days. What with baby boomers finding gray hairs in their combs, interest in staying healthy (read: young) has become an obsession. And vitamins at least appear to be The Magic Elixir. So vitamin hounds abound—but so do skeptics. Sometimes even the experts disagree (at least publicly).

Informal surveys at medical meetings across the country reveal what consumers have suspected all along—that an overwhelming majority of doctors and scientists are popping supplements themselves. Many are realists. They acknowledge that few women (or men, for that matter) eat the five daily servings of fruits and vegetables that medical studies have shown reduce the risk of heart disease, some kinds of cancer and many other ailments. So they recommend we get the nutrients

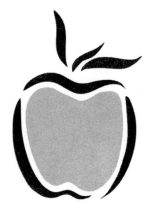

we need through supplements—and they're taking their own advice.

Whether or not you should be taking supplements depends on many factors—your diet, in particular. But to help you decide, here's a woman's guide to the latest vitamin research and expert recommendations. Highlighted are seven of the most important—and controversial—vitamins and minerals for women. Read on for the real scoop. Then decide for yourself whether you, too, should be taking supplements.

Beta-Carotene: Think Food

The claims: Supplemental beta-carotene may help combat cancer and heart disease.

The research: In the past decade, many study results have supported the cancer and heart disease claims. But a much-anticipated National Cancer Institute (NCI) study of beta-carotene and vitamin E use among 29,000 male smokers in Finland revealed that the supplements did not reduce study participants' rates for lung cancer. The consensus seems to be that, while beta-carotene is thought to be protective, it can't undo the damage from 20 years of cigarette smoking.

Gladys Block, Ph.D., professor of public health nutrition at the University of California at Berkeley, points out that the NCI study was flawed and that skeptics have dismissed the benefits of beta-carotene hastily. "Those clinical trials were done on people with precancerous conditions or on people at a very high risk of developing cancer," she says. "They don't really tell us about the *prevention* of disease."

Who can? Possibly, a team of researchers from Harvard University who are several years into a decade-long study on the effects of beta-

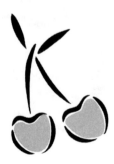

MULTIPLE CHOICE

*S*hould you swallow a supplement every morning? Or just on the days when your diet's a disaster? One way to tell is to keep track of what you eat for about a week, then compare your list with what follows. Every day, the average woman needs to consume:

- 2 to 3 servings of low-fat dairy products
- five to seven ounces of lean meat, poultry or fish
- 2 to 4 servings of fruit
- 3 to 5 servings of vegetables
- 6 to 11 servings of breads, cereals, rice or pasta

Most women don't meet these minimum requirements most days, says nutritionist Elizabeth Somer, R.D., author of *Nutrition for Women* and *Food and Mood*. "Most women fall short on two or three important nutrients every day," says Somer. "So I think it's smart—and safe—to take a multivitamin every day, as long as you steer clear of the ones that contain more than 100 percent of the Daily Value."

---

carotene supplements on heart disease and cancer in men. Preliminary results may be published next year.

The bottom line: Women should consume six milligrams—or 10,000 international units—of beta-carotene daily. A half-cup of boiled spinach, a cup of cantaloupe and half a carrot will give you a total of 16,500 international units. Supplement only if you don't get enough beta-carotene through your diet.

Vitamin C: More Than a Cold Cure

The claims: The late Nobel prize winner Linus Pauling, M.D., claimed for years that vitamin C can either help prevent or cure cancer and heart disease as well as help fight the common cold. And with current research apparently supporting some of his claims, the medical community has begun to agree. Many scientists now believe, for instance, that vitamin C can reduce the severity and duration of colds. And researchers are currently examining whether vitamin C protects against cancer and heart disease.

(continued on page 144)

SUPPLEMENTAL KNOWLEDGE

Here's a quick primer on each of the vitamins featured. Refer to it when planning your menus and when shopping for supplements.

Vitamin/Daily Value*	Food Sources
Beta-Carotene †	Cantaloupe, carrots, spinach, sweet potatoes and tomatoes.
Vitamin C 60 mg.	Broccoli, brussels sprouts, citrus fruits, guava, kiwifruit, red bell peppers and strawberries.
Vitamin D 400 IU	Egg yolks, fortified milk, liver, salmon and tuna canned in oil.
Vitamin E 30 IU	Almonds, avocados, broccoli, dried prunes, egg yolks, mayonnaise, safflower oil and wheat germ.
Folic Acid (Folate) 400 mcg.	Asparagus, brewer's yeast, broccoli, legumes, liver, orange juice, spinach and whole-wheat bread.
Calcium 1,000 mg.	Green leafy vegetables, milk and milk products, sardines with bones and tofu.
Iron 18 mg.	Eggs, green leafy vegetables, meat, tofu and whole grains.

*Daily Value is a term the U.S. Food and Drug Administration now uses in place of Recommended Daily Allowance, or RDA. These numbers simply represent the minimum recommended vitamin intake per day.

†There is no Daily Value set for beta-carotene, but 6 mg. is the equivalent of the recommended intake of vitamin A.

Functions

The body converts beta-carotene into Vitamin A, which aids the growth of bones, teeth and skin; prevents some eye disorders; ensures fertility and night vision and boosts the immune system.

Maintains healthy connective tissue, may help reduce the duration and severity of colds, appears to fight cataracts, speeds wound healing and reverses some types of male infertility.

Helps form bones and teeth and maintain their strength and is essential for the metabolism of calcium.

Protects tissues from toxins, may reduce the risk of heart disease, appears to prevent cataracts and boosts the immune system.

Makes new blood, muscle and skin cells; prevents neural-tube birth defects and may help prevent some blood disorders and cervical and colon cancer.

Maintains bone and tooth strength, muscle contraction, heartbeat, blood clotting and nerve function.

Helps maintain the immune system and carries oxygen.

The research: Supplemental vitamin C doesn't appear to protect against cancer, but eating an abundance of fruits and vegetables packed with vitamin C does. As for the heart-health claim, a ten-year study at the University of California, Los Angeles, School of Public Health revealed that people who consumed more than the Daily Value of vitamin C from food were less likely to die of heart disease than those who consumed less than the Daily Value. And their overall mortality rate was lower to boot.

The bottom line: In general, women should consume at least 60 milligrams of vitamin C a day—not hard to do when you consider that a four-ounce glass of orange juice contains 62 milligrams and a medium kiwifruit packs 75. If you're constantly stressed, or if you smoke or take birth control pills, consider boosting your vitamin C intake to at least 100 milligrams. To strengthen your immune system, you can safely supplement up to 1,000 milligrams daily.

Vitamin E: How Women Benefit

The claims: Although it definitely doesn't keep men from losing their sexual potency (sorry, that myth's been debunked), vitamin E is in the limelight again—this time for its apparent ability to fight heart disease and cataracts.

The research: In recent years, two Harvard University studies underscored the heart-health claim. Of the 87,245 women partici-

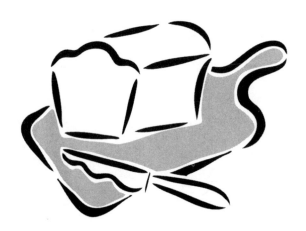

pants, those who supplemented their diets with at least 100 international units of vitamin E a day for two years or more cut their risk of suffering a heart attack by about 40 percent. As for E's effect on cataracts, several studies have indicated that daily supplements of vitamins E and C cut your risk of developing cataracts in half.

The bottom line: Shoot to consume 30 international units of vitamin E daily. Unfortunately, many foods high in E such as nuts and sunflower seeds are also high in fat. A few healthier options: spinach, sweet potatoes, asparagus and peaches.

If you'd like to take the doses used in most studies (up to 400 international units), you'll have to take a supplement. Opt for low-cost, synthetic versions of vitamin E—they're just as effective as the pricey "natural" forms—then be sure to take the pills with meals to improve their absorption.

Vitamin D: Go Easy on Supplements

The claims: Vitamin D may help protect against colon, rectal and possibly breast cancer.

The research: Several studies have shown that people who live in sunny climates develop fewer cases of colon, rectal and breast cancers than those who live in cloudy ones. (Exposure to the sun triggers the formation of vitamin D in the body.) But the mainstream medical community isn't ready to tout vitamin D as a cancer-reducer. The link between D and breast cancer will be fully explored by the Women's Health Initiative, one of the largest clinical vitamin trials ever conducted in this country. Results are expected in a few years.

The bottom line: It isn't tough to get 400 international units of vitamin D, the recommended intake, if you're regularly exposed to the sun, drink enough milk (100 international units per cup) and munch on fortified breakfast cereal (about 140 international units per half-cup).

If you're afraid you're falling short, reach for a multivitamin—just take care not to go overboard. Your body can excrete excess vitamin D from food but not from supplements. And taking more than 800 international units can be toxic, resulting in calcium deposits in your soft tissues and worse, permanent heart and kidney damage.

Folic Acid (Folate): Supercritical for Mom

The claims: An ample supply may help protect your unborn baby from severe spinal cord damage and lower your risk of cervical cancer.

The research: While folic acid plays a crucial role in making new blood, muscle and skin cells, many studies suggest that this B vitamin also greatly lowers a woman's risk of giving birth to a baby with anencephaly (a condition in which one or more vertebrae fail to develop completely, leaving a portion of the spinal cord exposed)—if it's consumed for up to two months before conception or in the first few weeks thereafter. And studies have shown that women who take folic acid supplements develop less precancerous cervical tissue than women who don't.

The bottom line: During your fertile years, you should consume 400 micrograms of folic acid a day. Most multivitamins will do the trick, as will a cup of orange juice (100 micrograms), a half-cup of red kidney beans (115 micrograms) and two spears of broccoli (180 micrograms).

Calcium: The Wisest Choices

The claims: Calcium may help protect women from osteoporosis later in life.

The research: A panel of experts convened by the National Institutes of Health (NIH) recently concluded that the Daily Value for calcium is too low, given the pivotal role the mineral plays in maintaining bone strength.

They recommend 1,200 milligrams a day for pregnant women over the age of 23, 1,000 milligrams a day for premenopausal women over the age of 25 and postmenopausal women taking estrogen, and 1,500 milligrams a day for postmenopausal women not taking estrogen.

The bottom line: Calcium is critical to maintaining bone strength, so make sure you get enough of it, either through supplements or your diet. Wise food choices include two ounces of reduced-fat Monterey Jack cheese (425 milligrams), an eight-ounce glass of skim milk (300 milligrams) and one cup of fortified orange juice (300 milligrams).

Iron: Needs Vary with Age

The claims: Supplemental iron helps cure fatigue.

The research: If you suffer from iron-deficiency anemia, supplemental iron will give you more energy (and often constipation). If you don't, some researchers not only refute iron's energizing claim, but link excess iron to heart attacks. They point to the fact that the incidence of heart attacks in women begins to catch up with the rate of heart attacks in men after women enter menopause. Why? Excess iron, they postulate. (We shed extra iron when we menstruate. But when we stop getting our periods regularly, iron builds up in our bodies and we suffer heart attacks more frequently.)

The bottom line: Given the wide variety of iron-rich foods such as dark green leafy vegetables, lean meat, legumes and fish, you should have no problem munching your way to the recommended 18 milligrams—especially if you eat foods high in vitamin C, which improves iron absorption. So, unless you're anemic or pregnant, you don't need to supplement.

What about the iron in a multivitamin? It's okay if you still menstruate. But after menopause, supplementing with iron is unnecessary and possibly harmful.

PART FOUR

Weight Control

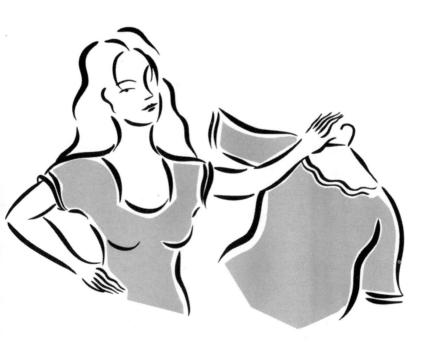

Why Women Need Food

Thinking it's "unlady-like" to satisfy your hunger will make you more than miserable. It might also make you fat.

When my sisters and brother and I were growing up, every so often during "dinner hour" my mom and dad would tell us the story of their first serious date.

"Your mother was the pickiest eater," my dad would recall, with a cavalier snicker. "I brought her to this fancy-shmansy restaurant, and she barely touched her prime rib."

To which my mom would proudly add, "So, of course, your father had to finish what was on my plate. I swear he had—and still has—a ferocious appetite!" Her eyes would widen, her lashes flutter.

As you've probably gathered from this exchange, Mom and Dad weren't talking just about food. Sex was an obvious undercurrent. Not the between-the-sheets variety, but sex in the gender sense. Me man, you woman. And although dinner-date dynamics may have evolved somewhat since the 1950s when my parents were courting, experts say that much remains the same.

When it comes to eating, men subconsciously think like Tarzan: Food is for survival. In addition, they link food and sex—the between-the-sheets kind. Basically, the hungrier, the hornier. And the hornier, well, the more manly.

Women's eating patterns are similarly gender-influenced. For us, food consumption is strongly connected to our womanliness . . . and requires restraint.

"Women have been taught for years to deny their hunger," explains Jennifer Stack, R.D., a nutritionist at New York University Medical Center in New York City. "And it's this denial that often leads to eating disaster."

Why? Because denial of any human need—food included—eventually triggers a knee-jerk reaction: the uncontrollable urge to overindulge. And that's when the cycle of unhealthy eating starts. Of course, the pressure to be feminine doesn't simply influence how much we eat. It also affects why, how and what we eat. Here's how gender plays a role in your eating habits and food preferences—and a few strategies for altering the behavior that may be sabotaging your diet.

The Scarlett O'Hara Effect

Feminism notwithstanding, wispy is still the ultimate in womanly—at least as far as the media is concerned. And if we're not extremely thin, society expects us to sustain ourselves on diet drinks and salad-only dinners. "It's simply not acceptable for women to have a hearty appetite or to be overweight," says Stack. "We're supposed to be slim and conscious of what we eat at all times."

Not so for men. "It's not as bad if a man has a ferocious appetite and is 35 pounds overweight," Stack says. "The excess weight almost gives him more power and presence." After all, modern-day Americans were raised on images of burly, manly men wolfing down hearty meals after a hard day's work. The women in these pictures simply watched their men chow down (after cooking for them, of course), smiling proudly.

A recent study conducted by Patricia Pliner, Ph.D., a social psychologist at the University of Toronto, supports this assertion. In her research, Dr. Pliner found that the women who ate little were received as more feminine than those who ate heartily, no matter how much they weighed. A man's projection of masculinity, however, wasn't affected at all by how much he ate. Pliner calls this phenomenon the Scarlett O'Hara effect—so named for the temperamental protagonist in *Gone with the Wind*, who gorged on buttermilk pancakes before attending a party so she wouldn't be tempted to eat in an "unladylike" fashion in public.

Experts say that it's this Scarlett O'Hara effect that accounts in part for the two genders' polar-opposite approaches and attitudes toward food. Men simply don't experience as much angst about eating as we women do. Women view edibles as evil, tempting and torturous—things to be reckoned with—while men view food as a right, something necessary for sustenance and satisfaction.

The Scarlett O'Hara factor also drives some women to engage in diet-destructive eating habits—call it a deprivation mentality. You're all too familiar with the scenario: You're at a party or on a dinner date.

You pass up dessert—then you pick at your date's. But you're still not satisfied because you feel shortchanged. So you go home, pull a carton of cookie dough ice cream out of the freezer (still wearing your coat) and start scarfing—alone.

"When we deny ourselves certain foods, we just end up hungry and more likely to binge or eat the wrong foods when we're alone," says Stack. That's why it's not only okay, it's downright healthful to openly indulge in generous portions and some so-called forbidden foods—even if you're overweight. If you don't, you ultimately do your psyche—and your waistline—a disservice. After all, it's basic human nature to want what we can't have.

Bottom line: Women need to avoid viewing any particular food as an absolute no-no. That done, we can teach ourselves to eat a variety of foods and perceive them as neither "good" nor "bad."

"You have to learn to be more honest with yourself about what you really want to eat," says Stack. "As long as you associate food with guilt, shame or disgust, you're never going to be able to approach eating in a healthy, positive way."

How—And What—Women Eat

Women graze. Men eat "real" meals. You figured as much, right? Now for the real news: When Marcia Pelchat, Ph.D., a research scientist at Monell Chemical Senses Center in Philadelphia, studied cravings among women and men, she found that, by and large, women tend to crave sweets more than entrées, and men crave entrées more than sweets.

In her study of about 100 men and women, Dr. Pelchat asked the participants about their cravings. She categorized their food preferences as either sweets (such as doughnuts, pies, candy and ice cream) or entrées (such as pizza, cheeseburgers and steaks). And she found that women craved the foods categorized as sweets at least twice as often as those considered entrées.

"We're not exactly sure why men and women tend to experience very different types of food cravings," says Dr. Pelchat. What we do know, however, is that if women by and large prefer sweets, odds are they're going to choose them as snacks between meals.

"While men are more apt to eat fewer, larger meals, women pick and snack," says Stack, "because they feel they shouldn't eat big meals." Now, nibbling isn't necessarily a bad thing, explains Stack. It's a sound strategy to eat many small meals throughout the day—as long as you satisfy your nutritional requirements and you aren't skipping meals.

Problem is, grazing can backfire—and often does—on women. We fall into the trap of what might be called reverse deprivation mentality. We're scared to death of overeating. But instead of depriving ourselves of certain "bad" foods altogether, we graze on small amounts of fatty treats or "fat-free" sweets that are calorie-laden. We figure, hey, a few Oreos never hurt anyone . . . and maybe they'll keep us from devouring an entire cake later. Unfortunately, guilt keeps us from eating a decent lunch or dinner, and then we're hungry less than an hour after we've eaten our meager meal—so we nibble even more.

It's this cyclic nibbling that's the problem. When we snack on potato chips and chocolate and then eat only a small portion of our spaghetti dinner, we appease—we don't please. And we're hungry constantly because we never really eat a full meal.

Of course, the multiple-meals approach can be a terrific one—when it's used within reason. Here's how to make it work: Since your system is ready for refueling every three or four hours, allow yourself a healthful yet tasty snack—such as pretzels, low-fat yogurt or fresh fruit—between breakfast and lunch, and then again between lunch and dinner. This way, your appetite won't be raging when mealtime approaches.

The trick to nibbling healthfully is to realize that a snack is just that—a snack. You still have to eat full, balanced meals. More important, if you do snack on an occasional bag of peanut M&Ms, don't do penance by cutting back on your lunch or dinner. Force yourself to eat full meals despite the indulgence. Just make sure that they're healthful.

—*Maureen Boland*

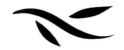

The Best Reason to Shed Those Pounds

Need more motivation? Consider this: Every lost pound helps reduce your risk of developing a host of ills.

Judging from the tidal waves of low-fat foods washing up on supermarket shelves and the multitude of health clubs popping up in cities, you'd think that America had become the land of the lean and the home of the fit.

Not by a long shot. In fact, one in three Americans—the highest number ever—is now seriously overweight, the National Center for Health Statistics in Bethesda, Maryland, has reported. Experts call obesity an epidemic—and it's one that's spawning major health problems in women. Heart disease, endometrial cancer and possibly breast cancer, high blood pressure, high cholesterol, immune system problems, gallstones, gout, diabetes, osteoarthritis, stroke and sleep apnea are all associated with overweight.

But do we really know what our healthiest weight is? How many of us are on target? And what are those who *are* on target doing differently from those who *aren't*?

To answer these questions, *Prevention* magazine surveyed women readers and got more than 10,000 responses. Here's an overview of the survey results.

The Frustrations of Fighting Fat

Frustration fairly leaped off the pages of the responses. Ninety percent of the respondents confessed they needed to lose weight (on average, 27 pounds). Only 14 percent described themselves as "well-toned," and just 7 percent said they were "very satisfied" with their bodies. More than half admitted they were "not very" or "not at all" satisfied.

But are so many female fat fighters really overweight, or do we just want to look slimmer?

In the opinion of top medical researchers and experts on obesity, many of the respondents had valid reasons for being concerned about their weight. "Slimmer is definitely healthier," observes William P. Castelli, M.D., medical director of the famed Framingham Heart Study, which followed 5,000 Massachusetts residents for 40 years to assess their risk for heart disease.

Fortunately, researchers are exploring ways to evaluate optimal body weight based on the latest research on weight-related health risks. Two approaches, used together, are emerging as the new "gold standard" for such evaluations: body mass index and waist/hip ratio.

An Index of Your Risk

Body mass index (BMI) is a ratio of height to weight. It's determined by a mathematical formula: First you divide your weight (in pounds) by your height (in inches) squared, then multiply the resulting number by 705. You should get a BMI that's somewhere between 19 and 30. But you don't have to do the calculations: Just see "Calculating Your BMI" on page 156.

Several large medical studies, involving thousands of people, have suggested that 21 to 22 is the optimal BMI. At this level, there are no weight-related health risks, according to Dr. Castelli. A BMI between 23 and 25 isn't ideal, some experts insist, but the excess risk for cancer and other weight-related diseases seems to be small at that level. Around a BMI of roughly 26, these health risks appear to rise, although scientists don't agree on exactly where to draw the line.

Most scientists do agree that a BMI over 27 increases risk for many people. But risk also depends on other factors, including waist/hip ratio, notes Jean Pierre Despres, Ph.D., associate director of the Lipid Research Center at Laval University in Sainte-Foy, Quebec.

Researchers have determined that the fat most associated with health risks is on the upper body—the abdomen and above—rather than on the thighs and hips. (A pattern of upper-body fat is often called central obesity.)

Some Hip Calculations

One way to judge whether you have too much upper-body fat is by measuring your waist (at the midpoint between your bottom rib and your hipbone) and your hips (at their widest point). Then divide the waist measurement by the hip measurement. The resulting number is your waist/hip ratio (WHR).

If your waist is 30 inches and your hips are 37 inches, for example, you would divide 30 by 37 to get a WHR of 0.81.

What's an ideal WHR? While scientists quibble over hundredths of a percent, most target 0.80 or less as desirable for both women and men.

CALCULATING YOUR BMI

To find your body mass index (BMI), locate your height in the left column. (If you've lost inches over the years, use your peak adult height.) Move across the chart to the right until you hit your approximate weight. Then follow that column down to the corresponding BMI number at the bottom of the chart.

If your BMI is 21 to 22: Super! Your BMI is right where it should be.

If your BMI is 23 to 25: At this BMI, the risk of developing weight-

Height	Body Weight in Pounds					
4'10"	91	96	100	105	110	115
4'11"	94	99	104	109	114	119
5'0"	97	102	107	112	118	123
5'1"	100	106	111	116	122	127
5'2"	104	109	115	120	126	131
5'3"	107	113	118	124	130	135
5'4"	110	116	122	128	134	140
5'5"	114	120	126	132	138	144
5'6"	118	124	130	136	142	148
5'7"	121	127	134	140	146	153
5'8"	125	131	138	144	151	158
5'9"	128	135	142	149	155	162
5'10"	132	139	146	153	160	167
5'11"	136	143	150	157	165	172
6'0"	140	147	154	162	169	177
BMI	19	20	21	22	23	24

This technique isn't very reliable for women who are very thin or very overweight. But in most cases, it can prove very predictive of cardiovascular disease risk.

"Central obesity is turning out to be the most lethal risk factor associated with excess body weight," says Dr. Castelli. That's because upper-body fat is strongly correlated with visceral fat, which is fat that's packed around our internal organs.

While most of the research on the health risks of upper-body fat

---

related ailments like cancer and heart disease seems to be small. Still, you may want to lower your BMI to a more healthful level.

If your BMI is 26: At this BMI, weight-related health risks appear to rise, but experts aren't exactly sure by how much.

If your BMI is 27 or above: Most experts agree that a BMI over 27 increases the risk of developing weight-related ailments. Consult your doctor about your weight-loss options.

119	124	129	134	138	143	148	153
124	128	133	138	143	148	153	158
128	133	138	143	148	153	158	163
132	137	143	148	153	158	164	169
136	142	147	153	158	164	169	174
141	146	152	158	163	169	175	180
145	151	157	163	169	174	180	186
150	156	162	168	174	180	186	192
155	161	167	173	179	186	192	198
159	166	172	178	185	191	197	204
164	171	177	184	190	197	203	210
169	176	182	189	196	203	209	216
174	181	188	195	202	207	215	222
179	186	193	200	208	215	222	229
184	191	199	206	213	221	228	235
25	**26**	**27**	**28**	**29**	**30**	**31**	**32**

has been done with men, more research with women is beginning. Researchers at the University of Miami School of Medicine and the University of Minnesota School of Public Health in Minneapolis, for example, examined data on 32,898 healthy women ages 55 to 69. In a four-year period, there were nearly three times as many heart disease deaths among women with the highest WHR (over 0.86) as among women with the lowest.

A high WHR has also been associated with diabetes, hypertension, breast and endometrial cancers and high cholesterol.

Dr. Castelli is one of several scientists who believe that WHR is even more important than BMI in predicting risk. "If someone has a healthy body mass index but a high WHR, it is important to try to bring that WHR down," he explains. "Someone with a higher BMI but a low WHR might not be quite as bad off."

Overweight or Overfat?

According to weight-control experts, some women may be confusing overweight with overfat. If you're in the "optimal" range, you may not need to lose pounds. But even so, you may need to lose fat and improve muscle tone.

Along with BMI and WHR, muscle tone does have relevance to health risks and weight. After all, scientists agree that the danger of overweight generally is not from heavy bones or muscles; it's from excess fat.

Exact standards don't exist for how much body fat a person can carry without increasing risk, but at the Cooper Aerobics Center in Dallas, they aim for 18 to 22 percent of total weight as optimal for women, slightly higher than for men.

Unfortunately, it's not easy to determine percentage of body fat. There are several ways to go about it, from pinching skin folds with calipers to bioelectric impedance (running a mild current through the body to measure resistance) to underwater weighing. These methods are not widely available outside health clubs or specialists' offices and are not always reliable.

But you can often eyeball it, according to Joan Marie Conway, Ph.D., research chemist at the U.S. Department of Agriculture (USDA)

Human Nutrition Research Center in Beltsville, Maryland. An easy way to judge whether you're overfat is by looking in a mirror, she explains. If, despite good BMI and WHR numbers, you look flabby, you probably are. And you'd do well to embark on an exercise regimen that burns fat and tones muscle.

Through all the weighing and measuring, it's important not to get too hung up on the scale or measuring tape, she adds. "You could never use one number to tell someone their risk for disease," says Dr. Conway.

Other doctors agree. "There are other factors, like family history, good and bad health habits like smoking and exercising or personal health risks like high cholesterol, low high-density lipoprotein (HDL) cholesterol (the good kind) or high blood pressure to consider, too," says Dr. Despres. "People with more risk factors must be more careful of their weight."

Clearly, finding your perfect weight for health is not yet a precise science. But it's safer to err on the side of slender, says Dr. Castelli. "You may be on the borderline today, but where are you going to be five years from now? Get in the habit of controlling your weight before you have a problem, not after."

Flexing Your Way to Success

Many of the women who responded to the *Prevention* survey found that weight loss wasn't so hard. The toughest challenge, many said, was keeping the weight off. For them, exercise was an important factor. Forty-eight percent of the women with optimal weight were in the habit of exercising four or more times weekly.

Based on the experience of these women, here are some exercise tips that will help you go the extra mile.

Stretch your exercise time. "It's known that the only way to maintain weight loss forever is to increase the amount of physical activity you do," says Miriam Nelson, Ph.D., research scientist at the USDA Human Nutrition Research Center on Aging at Tufts University in Boston.

Indeed, though women of optimal weight were no more active in their daily lives than overweight respondents, they did participate in more intentional exercise. In the optimal weight group, most women said their workout sessions lasted between a half-hour and an hour. Severely overweight women most commonly report the shortest exercise sessions—less than 20 minutes.

Go for pleasure. To exercise consistently, of course, you must find a form of exercise (or a combination of exercises) that you actually enjoy. "It needs to be something people like and feel they can continue doing indefinitely," says James O. Hill, Ph.D., associate director of the Center for Human Nutrition at the University of Colorado Health Sciences Center in Denver.

For people at risk from overweight, Dr. Despres recommends walking, walking, walking. The risk of injury is lower than for many other exercises. "We have shown that this is an excellent form of exercise to decrease excess abdominal fat and the complications associated with it," he explains.

"Even if you don't lose a lot of weight, your risk profile will improve with a brisk 45-minute walk four or five days a week," he continues. "If you don't exercise that much, you won't burn enough fat to get the substantial improvement in your risk profile that you'd see with that program."

Weight up. The *Prevention* survey also revealed that women who have optimal body weight do more strength training. Thirty-five percent of those in the optimal group were hefting small weights or using resistance machines to strengthen muscle, compared with 14 percent or fewer of those in heavier groups.

Why is strength training so important to maintaining healthy body weight? "Large muscle mass helps burn calories," Dr. Nelson explains. "More muscle means a faster metabolism." That's because muscle requires more oxygen and more calories to sustain itself than fat does. And strength training is more effective than aerobic exercise at building and maintaining muscle.

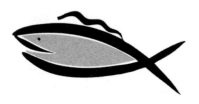

What about Diet?

Of course, low-fat eating goes hand-in-hand with exercise. "When you combine strength training and aerobic exercise with sensible eating, you'll look trimmer, feel more fit and be able to eat more," observes Wayne Westcott, Ph.D., strength consultant to the YMCA, IDEA: International Association of Fitness Professionals and the American Council on Exercise.

But how do you find comfortable limits without going on a diet? Here are the strategies recommended by experts.

Learn your body signals. Have you lost the ability to distinguish between emotional and physiological hunger and just plain boredom? If you have, your best bet to dump those unnecessary pounds and maintain a stable weight is to tap into what your body wants and doesn't want, says Steven C. Strauss, M.D., an internist in New York City specializing in nutrition and weight control and author of *The Body Signal Secret.*

As you eat, become aware of how you feel when you're satisfied, when you're full and when you're stuffed, Dr. Strauss advises. Then decide to stop eating whenever you hit the full mark. "If you eat only when you're hungry and stop when you're satisfied, your body will reach its optimal weight," says Dr. Strauss.

Multiply meals, shrink portions. If you're a devotee of three meals a day, you may be consuming more calories than you need at those meals and storing the rest as fat. That's because "your body can only use a certain amount of calories at a time to function," says nutritionist Debra Waterhouse, R.D., author of *Outsmarting the Female Fat Cell.* Eating four or five mini-meals a day will prevent the problem.

Break the morning fast. "Never, ever eliminate breakfast," says Dr. Strauss. "Try to eat grains, fresh fruits and vegetables."

If you usually start your day with just a cup of coffee, your metabolism is probably sluggish, burning fewer calories than it should from subsequent meals. Since our bodies burn calories at a slower rate while we sleep, breakfast acts as reveille for our metabolism. In fact, a study at George Washington University in Washington, D.C., showed a metabolic increase of 3 to 4 percent above average in morning eaters.

Fill up on fiber. "High-fiber foods promote a feeling of fullness more readily than low-fiber meals," says Dr. Strauss. So "you feel more satisfied with less food."

Try hot oatmeal for breakfast, vegetarian chili for lunch and five-bean casserole for dinner. Aim for 35 grams of fiber a day.

Forgo excess fat. Fat calories are much harder to burn than calories from carbohydrates and proteins. They're also easily converted to body fat. That's why you should keep fat calories to 25 percent or less of your daily diet.

How? First, avoid deep-fried or breaded and fried foods. Instead, go for broiled, grilled or baked fish and skinless chicken. Use a non-stick pan or oil sprays or chicken broth for sautéeing. Try evaporated skim milk as a substitute for whole milk or cream.

Also, be sure to trim the fat off all meats before cooking. And for sweet treats, reach for fruit and nonfat products. Or at least read labels to check how much fat is in each product. "If the percentage of fat is greater than 15 percent, you may want to replace that item on the shelf," says Dr. Strauss.

50 Little Ways to Lose a Lot of Weight

Not ready to plunge into a diet? No problem: These bite-size tips can pay off big when you step on the scale.

Imagine giving in to a craving and feeling *good* about it . . . getting through a binge without completely undoing your diet . . . learning to love a daily workout.

Dream on, you say? Think again: You can turn these "fantasies" into realities. What's more, these little steps, and others like them, can propel your weight-loss efforts a long, long way.

Prevention magazine asked some of the country's leading weight-loss experts in nutrition, physiology and psychology for their best tips on how to help you break the weight-loss barrier, whether you're trying to lose your first pound or your 50th. The keys: planning, attitude, exercise (of course) and brain work.

Be a Woman with a Plan

You've probably heard the old saying, "failing to plan is planning to fail." And many of our weight-loss experts agree that planning, in a variety of forms, is what makes the difference between a successful weight-loss strategy and one that never gets legs.

If you set goals and don't make plans to meet them, you'll fall back into the same eating and exercise patterns you're used to. Many of the suggestions we got from the experts are about taking the time to set goals and plan each and every day for the ways you'll meet them.

Crush mall cravings. If you're going to the mall and you know you're going to smell pizza or cinnamon buns that will make your mouth water, be prepared. Eat before you go out so you won't be as temptable. And don't shop until you drop. Plan a snack that fits into your calorie/fat-gram plan. Either carry it with you or know just where to purchase it.

Learn the ten-minute rule. If a craving hits for a hot-fudge sundae and it's not in your plan for the day, distract yourself for at least ten minutes. In most cases, the craving will pass. Meditate, call a friend, go for a walk. If after ten minutes your craving hasn't subsided, you may be truly hungry. Look for a healthy low-fat snack.

Plan to eat at home. That's one of the few places where you really know what you're putting in your mouth. But if your lifestyle demands eating out, or occasional fast fixes, plan for them! Most fast-food eateries supply handy pamphlets describing in detail the caloric and fat content of their menu items. Collect these pamphlets and analyze them for your favorite low-fat meals. Then when you have to make a stop, you know just what to order, without even looking at the choices.

For more-expensive restaurants, call ahead and ask what's low-fat and low-calorie on the menu. Many places will prepare a special meal if you give them notice. Poring over the menu when you get there puts too many tempting images in your mind.

Don't plan on willpower. Physiology always beats out psychology. In other words, hunger beats out self-control. To get around that, try to plan your day so you aren't forced to use self-control. It's the old "don't-go-grocery-shopping-on-an-empty-stomach" idea. Expand that concept to your whole day. Don't blame yourself for lack of willpower after an indulgence. Just evaluate how you can plan better to avoid it in the future.

Keep a food diary. Choose a way to keep track of what and when you eat every day. You may choose to track fat grams, calories, exchanges—the method is up to you. It seems that just keeping track is what helps people cut back, not brutal honesty or a foolproof memory. In fact, when starting out, don't even try to make any changes. Just get an idea of what it is you're eating every day to maintain the weight that you are.

Revamp Your Attitude

Changing your lifestyle means changing your attitude toward a lot of things. You set new priorities and you learn new likes and dislikes. Be ready to incorporate new ideas to help you change old habits.

Set goals and priorities. Spend some time working out your goals on paper. It's important that they're not vague. It's also important that they're reasonable. If you're not sure if your weight-loss goals are reasonable, seek out a qualified health professional to give you an objective perspective.

Take stock of your shelves. Look through your pantry and your refrigerator and get rid of any foods that don't fit in with your new goals for weight control. Donate them to a local charity and then restock with foods that fit in with your new meal plans. There are lots of new foods on the market that can help you cut calories and fat without sacrificing taste. You can change just about any favorite high-fat meal into a low-fat version.

Read about it. Read a lot about weight loss, diet, nutrition and exercise. Not only may you find it motivating and inspiring, you should also have more ideas to help you tailor a program that meets your needs. One study has shown that people who take the bull by the horns and design their own programs are the most successful at losing weight and keeping it off.

Focus on maintenance. There is a possibility that weight cycling (losing, gaining, losing) is linked to bad health. However, a fear of weight cycling should not deter anyone from attempting to reach a healthy weight. Lately, a popular theory has been that most people who lose weight eventually gain it back, and then some. This may fast become a self-fulfilling prophecy. The problem is, most studies on people losing weight are done in clinical or hospital settings. And often those people comply with a special weight-reduction program as long as they are active (or captive) participants. When they go back home, they go back to old habits. People who design their own programs at home often are much more successful at maintaining their weight losses. Just look around you. Chances are you know people who've lost weight and kept it off for years. And you thought they were an exception to the rule!

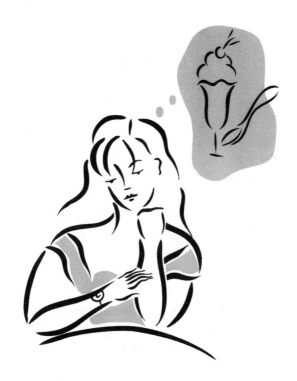

Know serving sizes. Counting fat grams is not enough. Studies show that people can still gain weight eating a low-fat diet. They may load up on low-fat foods. It's important to watch the total amount of food you eat. Portion control is essential. The American Heart Association puts out a pamphlet, "The American Heart Association Diet," that gives tips on determining portions. Call 1-800-242-8721 to order the free brochure. Spend some time measuring out portions and seeing what they look like on the plate so you can judge when to stop serving yourself. Do you really know what a cup of spaghetti looks like?

Use the one-to-one rule. Use fat-free and sugar-free products, but use them wisely. A one-to-one substitution is best. In other words, substitute one fat-free Twinkie for one regular Twinkie. Don't kid yourself into thinking you can eat two or three because they're low in fat. Sugary calories add up to fat in your body.

No food outlaws. Don't feel you have to ban chocolate or any other favorite foods. If you watch your portions and/or your calories, you can find room for any food. Depriving yourself may set you up for bingeing.

Working Out: Get off Your "But"

To lose weight and keep it off, exercise has to become a regular part of your everyday life, no ifs, ands or "but I don't have the time" about it. If you don't have time for exercise, you don't have the means to permanent weight control. Once you realize it's the only way out, you may begin to find the time you need.

Team up with your doctor. In a recent survey by the President's Council on Physical Fitness and Sports, respondents said they thought they would be more motivated to exercise if their doctors told them to. If you feel like you fall into that category, find a doctor who will encourage you. Although there are no studies to confirm the results for weight loss, studies have shown that doctors' encouragement definitely helped people quit smoking.

Learn to love resistance training. Increasing or maintaining your lean body mass is a crucial component in the weight-loss game plan. The more muscle you have, the more calories you burn, whether

SNIFF AWAY POUNDS

Sniffing certain scents may help people to curb their appetites or increase their exercise, says Alan Hirsch, M.D., neurologist and director of the Smell and Taste Research Foundation in Chicago.

In one study, men and women on exercise bikes were able to burn more calories during the same three-minute interval when they sniffed certain scents. Women perked up for strawberries and men for the smell of baking bread. (Dr. Hirsch used chemical representatives—not natural odors—in his study.)

In another study, men and women sniffed banana, peppermint or green-apple-scented inhalers whenever they felt the urge to eat. On average they lost 4.7 pounds a month, even though they were told not to change their usual eating patterns. The more people sniffed, the more weight they lost.

Dr. Hirsch doesn't think these particular scents are special, just that most people like them. And he doesn't know whether the smell short-circuited their appetites or if grabbing the inhaler just reminded them not to eat.

you're exercising or sleeping. Weight lifting is a unique exercise in that it enhances lean body mass. While aerobic exercises, such as walking, jogging and bicycling, are important for fat burning, they don't substantially increase lean body mass. And as we age, that lean body mass tends to decrease.

Weight training should be done two or three times a week, unless you target different muscle groups on different days, in which case you can work out more often.

Learn the 80 percent solution. To increase muscle mass you need to do high-intensity weight training. That means finding the weight that you can lift about 8 to 12 times and no more. At that rate, you're lifting about 80 percent of your capacity. (If you lift a weight 25 times without tiring, you tone your muscles, but you don't increase muscle mass.) It's fine to start with lighter weights to train your muscles to get ready for heavier work.

Walk and weight train. To lose weight, most people need to commit to at least 45 minutes to an hour of low-intensity endurance training, like brisk walking, almost every day. So if you're lifting weights one day, you should still try to get your walk in. (We know it's hard.) Unless you're a bodybuilder who needs to maximize her output in one area, you can do both and enhance your weight-loss program without harming your body. Try doing one in the morning and the other in the late afternoon or evening, to avoid fatigue.

Try dumbbells. To weight train you don't have to buy a membership in a fitness center or buy expensive home gyms. To start out, buy a $20 set of barbells with instructions, and work out at home. You can see how you like it without a big investment. If you're unsure how to use your barbells, seek instruction from a certified health and fitness instructor at your local YMCA or fitness club. As you progress, you may find fitness centers great places to meet lifting buddies or to learn more about your new sport.

Keep a journal. Just like food diaries, exercise journals help keep you motivated to do what it is you want to do. Keep one for weight lifting to show your progress and keep another for aerobic activity. If you're not keen on spending a full hour exercising continuously, remember, it's the sum total of exercise you do in one day that matters most, not whether you do it all at the same time. Four 15-minute sessions are as effective at burning calories as one continuous hour.

Find some good videos. Ask your friends if they have any favorite workout videos. Keep a collection around so you can vary your workout from time to time to avoid boredom. You can even borrow videos from your local public library to keep things interesting. Instead of a walk outside, go inside and try step-aerobics or polka or country-western dancing. Just don't try to do the whole tape the first day out. Ease into it, or you may be too sore to get out of bed the next day.

Break Through Old Baggage

Many of our barriers to weight loss are mental and emotional ones. While some people may need counseling to break through their weight-loss wall, others can use simple mental techniques to help institute healthy habits.

Visualize your goal and how you'll get there. Spend some time every day visualizing yourself at your ideal and realistic weight. See yourself doing the behaviors you need to do to obtain the results you want. Use all your senses to imagine yourself enjoying a delicious apple if you need to eat more fruit. Or vividly imagine how you'll feel on a brisk morning walk.

De-stress to fight fat. Stress might have an impact on the way your body metabolizes fat. In addition to that, you may eat more when you're feeling pressured. So find ways, such as walking or meditation, to reduce the effects of stress. Do whatever you need to do to keep your life in balance.

Stop negative self-talk. Become aware of all the little ways you sabotage yourself through your thoughts. We all occasionally carry on internal dialogues that can stand in the way of success. Catch yourself saying "I'll never lose weight" or "I hate to exercise" and replace those thoughts with more positive ones.

Learn relapse prevention. It's normal to relapse—to go back to being a slug or eating high-fat foods—for a day, a week or even more. That's part of the pattern of change and growth, not the end of your weight-loss efforts. When it happens, use it as a learning experience. Ask yourself what was going on in your life when the relapse occurred. Family pressures? Work stress? Your sister Mary offering you homemade chocolate cake? Then try to make plans to meet those relapse triggers more successfully in the future.

Get more sleep. Many people work too hard and get too little sleep. We may even eat to compensate for our lack of sleep. It may give us a quick boost, but we end up storing the extra calories as fat. When you need to work long hours, try walks or showers rather than candy bars to boost your energy.

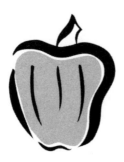

Two Dozen Ways to De-fat Your Diet

Think you know every fat-trimming trick in the book?
Wait until you try these tips.

*Y*ou want to de-fat your diet. Really you do. But if going low-fat means you have to turn your favorite sweet, creamy, cheesy comfort foods into so much cardboard, you'll keep your fettucine Alfredo and chocolate chip cookies, thanks.

If that about sums up your attitude toward low-fat cooking, here's some delicious help from some of the most fat-conscious sources around: chefs in the ritziest restaurants, the private cooks of health-fanatical celebs and best-selling cookbook authors. The result—25 easy fat-trimming techniques you most likely haven't heard before. You're sure to be enticed to try at least a few of the pro tips that follow and make some of them part of your regular fat-trimming repertoire.

Fat-Slashed Flash-Frying

Know your butter subs. Everyone knows there are stand-ins for butter and oil in sautéing. But selecting the *right* substitute is the secret to success.

- Use four tablespoons of wine or stock per one tablespoon of oil in the original recipe. You'll save 14 grams of fat and up to 42 calories.
- Use red wine in tomato dishes (to sauté garlic and onions for pasta sauce, for instance).
- Substitute a fruity white or blush wine for olive oil when preparing light dishes such as mild fish. Avoid dry white wines, which leave a metallic taste.
- When in doubt, chicken stock is a good, all-purpose stand-in for olive oil in almost any dish.

Pound out fat. This may sound like work, but the couple of extra minutes it adds to sautéing chicken and firm-flesh fish, such as tuna or swordfish, is well worth it: Use a pastry brush to lightly "paint" two pieces of parchment paper with a little olive oil. Place the food between the sheets of paper and pound gently with a rolling pin. This leaves a thin coat of oil, just enough to prevent sticking, and because the food is flattened, it will cook quickly without drying out.

Make your own (nearly) no-stick pan. Place a sturdy sauté pan on the stove over high heat. When the pan starts to smoke, rub a teaspoon of salt along the inside. (Careful—the pan will be hot!) This makes the pan less absorbent, so that when oil is used, it won't soak into the pan, necessitating the addition of more oil during cooking. Season your pan often—at least once a week if possible.

Sprinkle away fat. Sprinkle veggies with about half a teaspoon of salt during the first stage of sautéing: This brings out the liquid in the vegetable, so you can use much less oil.

Luscious, Low-Fat Desserts

Use fruit, not fat. Purees of fresh or dried fruit are standard stand-ins for fat in baked goods, but certain ones work best in certain recipes. In most cases, you can replace up to seven-eighths of the butter or shortening called for in a traditional recipe with one of the substitutes below: Half a cup of butter has 91 grams of fat, while fruit purees have none, and only a fraction of the calories.

- Fresh fruit purees, such as mashed bananas and applesauce, work best in light cakes and muffins.
- Make raisin "paste" to replace the butter or oil in dense, chewy cookies, like oatmeal or chocolate chip. Mash raisins in a food processor until they have the same consistency as butter.
- Pureed prunes are the best substitute for butter in chocolate treats like brownies.

Choose cake flour. Bake fat-reduced cakes with cake flour instead of the all-purpose variety; this flour will help keep cakes light and airy.

Slash fat with syrup. Light or dark corn syrup can fill in for some of the fat in desserts. Substitute one tablespoon of corn syrup per two tablespoons of fat. You'll save 28 grams of fat and 200 calories for every couple of tablespoons of fat omitted.

Eschew eggs for gelatin. Gelatin can replace eggs in desserts such as mousses and doesn't interfere with flavor. Use one tablespoon dissolved gelatin per two cups total liquid; you'll trim five grams of fat and about 60 calories per egg left out.

Creamy-Yet-Creamless Sauces and Soups

Take stock. The base for many cream sauces is a *roux*—a sauté of butter and flour. To make a nearly fat-free but just as flavorful roux, substitute chicken stock for the butter: Over low heat, mix a couple of tablespoons each chicken stock and flour and cook, stirring constantly, until thick and lightly colored. A white sauce made this way will have 16 fewer grams of fat and 100 fewer calories than one made with a butter-based roux.

Blend away fat. Pureed parsnips can fill in for some or all of the cream in many soups, and taste more like cream than other vegetable stand-ins like potatoes. Plus, they're fat-free and low-cal—only 60 calories per half-cup. Half a cup of cream weighs in at 44 grams of fat and 410 calories.

Leaner Greens

Create your own croutons. Instead of using oily, homemade croutons, break up fat-free flavored rice cakes to toss in salads. You'll pare as many as 16 grams of fat and save over 100 calories per half-cup of rice cakes.

Cheat on the cheese. To make a low-fat blue cheese dressing, warm plain yogurt and blue cheese for a minute or two on low. Heating intensifies the flavor of the cheese so you can use a tiny amount—about a tablespoon per four servings—and still get a full-flavored dressing. You'll save 15 grams of fat and around 120 calories.

Pare down your Caesar. A puree of six cloves of roasted garlic, half a cup of basil leaves, two to three tablespoons of honey and a quarter-cup of balsamic vinegar tastes remarkably like the conventional egg-oil-anchovy dressing. You'll save eight grams of fat and 60 calories.

High-Flavor, Low-Fat Mix-Ins

Go nuts for less fat. Replace nuts like walnuts or pecans with chopped chestnuts or water chestnuts (in chicken salad, for instance). You'll trim about five grams of fat and up to 40 calories per tablespoon of nuts.

Oust olives. Capers fill in nicely for olives; they add sharp, salty flavor, but with a significant fat savings. One tablespoon of capers per quarter-cup of olives should do it—and you'll be down four grams of fat and about 30 calories. Just remember to rinse the capers before using.

Fat-Trimming Tofu Tricks

Hold the mayo. Blend tofu with a dried dip mix (such as onion or garlic) and spread on bread in place of mayonnaise. Per two tablespoons, you'll save 19 grams of fat and 200 calories. If you're watching your sodium intake, look for low-sodium dip mixes.

Chuck the cheese. Smoked tofu, available in health food stores and some supermarkets, is an excellent substitute for smoked cheese on pizza, pasta and in sandwiches. Best of all, an ounce of tofu has only 20 calories and one gram of fat, compared to the 115 calories and nine grams of fat in an ounce of cheese.

Wrap It Up

Cooking *en papillote*—wrapping foods in parchment paper or foil—is a standard fat-saving trick. The food steams in added liquids, such as wine, fruit juices or marinades, as well as in its own cooking juices, so there's no need to add oil or butter. The unique wrappers that follow impart flavors of their own to food. Plus, you can eat some of the wrappers—no paper or foil to futz with.

Try a healthy husk. Stuff veggies, seafood and herbs into moistened corn husks, tie closed with a thin strip of the husk, then steam, bake or grill.

Wrap it up. Roll bite-size pieces of seafood and veggies in flour tortillas and steam.

Invent veggie packages. Wrap fish in thin slices of daikon radish or turnip and poach in a mixture of wine and ginger juice (squeeze chunks of ginger in a garlic press). To make a fat-free sauce, reduce the poaching liquid with julienne carrots and cilantro.

Bring home the (Italian) bacon. To enjoy the rich flavor of smoky meats for less fat, wrap a thin slice or two of pancetta (Italian bacon) around a chicken breast or lean cut of meat and bake. Pancetta contains only one gram of fat and 21 calories per half-ounce to regular bacon's seven grams of fat and 82 calories.

A Trio of Miscellaneous Fat Trimmers

Broil on branches. Rather than coating the grill or broiler with oil to prevent sticking, dip several sprigs of a sturdy herb such as rosemary, oregano, thyme or sage in olive oil, squeeze off the excess oil and layer the herbs between broiler and poultry, fish or meat.

Make grilled-veggie mosaics. *Terrines*—layers of vegetables and/or meats—are typically "bound" with cream-based mousses. For a virtually fat-free terrine, layer slices of roasted or grilled veggies in a pan and pour reduced chicken or beef stock over them. The stock congeals as it cools, holding the terrine together. Sliced into squares, this low-fat terrine costs 2 grams of fat and 60 calories, versus 29 grams of fat and 185 calories in a regular terrine.

Perfect your pasta. Rather than adding oil to thick, low-moisture pasta sauces (like veggie- or cheese-based toppings), juice up the pasta. For one pound of pasta: Drain cooked noodles, return to pan with one cup of chicken stock and cook until the stock is reduced by about half. Then add the sauce. You'll save 40 grams of fat and 340 calories per quarter-pound serving.

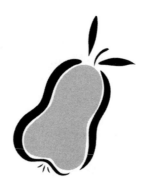

PART FIVE

Body-Shaping

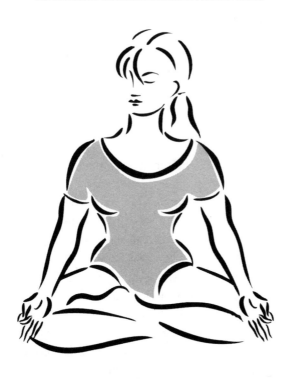

Your Fat-Blasting Action Plan

Here's one diet expert's winning strategies to help you shed pounds and keep them off.

*H*ave you become a certifiable yo-yo? We mean an ever-fluctuating dieter. Summertime you're slim, wintertime you're plump. After a weekend of visiting with friends (read: eating with them), the waistband of your favorite pair of jeans feels as if it's cutting off your circulation, and only after a week of intense dieting does it relax.

It's time to face facts: Losing weight requires more than emergency measures like crash dieting. Research has shown that the best predictor for maintaining weight loss is exercise. "By reducing sedentary behavior and increasing activity through planned exercise and everyday habits, weight loss will come—and stay—for good," says diet expert James O. Hill, Ph.D., associate director of the Center for Human Nutrition at the University of Colorado Health Sciences Center in Denver.

Burn, Baby, Burn

Dr. Hill's approach is simple: While maintaining your caloric intake, increase activity in three key areas of your life. "During the day, you're either inactive, taking part in daily activities or engaging in some planned exercise," says Dr. Hill. "By targeting those three areas with small changes, together they can have an enormous impact in terms of weight loss."

Let's say you want to lose six pounds and keep the weight off for good. "In order to lose that weight, you would have to keep your calorie intake constant and burn off roughly 150 extra calories of energy each and every day," says Dr. Hill. "You would then look at those three areas and figure out where to burn those 150 calories."

First, take a look at the amount of time you spend sitting, watch-

WHAT? NO DIET?

*Y*ou may have noticed that something is glaringly missing from Dr. Hill's permanent-weight-loss strategy: diet. That's the good news. This program focuses only on exercise; the weight-loss results to come don't factor in the extra benefit to be gained from a healthy low-fat diet.

"Whatever dietary changes you make are simply an added bonus to the weight-loss mix," says Dr. Hill. By cutting down on fatty snacks and choosing instead fresh fruits, vegetables, pastas and grains as your main food sources, you may in time even surpass Dr. Hill's peak goal of 25 pounds. We aren't talking deprivation, either—only sensible diet changes and substitutions.

ing TV or napping—your sedentary time. "By replacing 30 to 40 minutes of inactivity with some leisurely walking, you can increase the amount of energy burned that day by 40 to 60 calories," says Dr. Hill.

Next, analyze your routine activities—the time you spend in motion, such as the chores of raking leaves, vacuuming, digging in the garden and running errands on foot. "By increasing the amount of daily activities you do—say taking the stairs instead of the elevator or walking at lunch instead of reading the newspaper—you can easily burn off another extra 50 calories," says Dr. Hill.

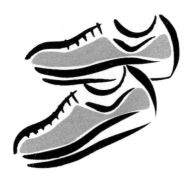

Finally, target your daily planned exercise. By adding an extra 15 minutes to your evening stroll, bam! You've peeled off another 50-plus calories, putting you over the top for your 150-calorie goal. But be patient—weight loss may take a while.

That's just one example of how to follow Dr. Hill's plan for permanent weight loss. By increasing activity in these ways, it may help you to permanently lose as much as 25 pounds.

Now you can come up with your own action plan, based on the doctor's novel approach: Just spread the work around however you like. A little less sitting around here, a few household chores there and some extra walking or jogging at night. "By spreading it around, the commitment isn't as challenging and you're much more likely to succeed," says Dr. Hill.

The Key to Success: Be Realistic

Whether your weight-loss goal is 5 pounds or 25, check the chart below to determine exactly what you will need to do in the calorie-burning department. Once you pick a realistic goal, decide where this calorie deficit can best fit into your life. "Remember, you don't adapt to this program, it adapts to you," says Dr. Hill. But be realistic. If you have 25 pounds to lose, don't start off trying to burn the 600 calories

---

LOSE WEIGHT THROUGH EXERCISE

You can lose weight without dieting. Below are the number of calories you would need to burn each day—and how much time it might take—to achieve your weight-loss goal.

Weight-Loss Goal (in Pounds)	Calories to Burn Each Day through Exercise	Estimated Time (Weeks)
5 to 6	150	17
10 to 12	300	20
15 to 18	450	20
20 to 25	600	21

needed each day, especially if you have been sedentary for a long time. "Start with a goal of 150 calories per day. Then slowly build on your calorie deficit, so in time you are burning enough to reach your goal," says Dr. Hill. The weight-loss goals Dr. Hill lists are to be achieved over one year's time.

Be aware that when you burn more calories than usual, you may compensate for some of that burn-off by eating more. "The weight-loss goals listed are based on the assumption that you may compensate in calories," says Dr. Hill. Translation: If you burn an extra 300 calories a day, you can eat a few extra calories and still hit your goal. But keep in mind that you'll reach your goal more quickly if you don't eat more.

It's possible to reach the first two goals of 5 to 6 pounds and 10 to 12 pounds through exercise alone. But once you shoot for 15 pounds and beyond, exercise alone may not be enough to help you reach your goal. It may also help to adhere to a low-fat diet.

Part I: Stretch beyond Your Sedentary Mode

"Sedentary" is a nice word for doing nothing. At rest or sitting you expend a paltry 50 to 70 calories per hour. "Some people who are sedentary during the day at work or at home and then watch television at night can rack up eight hours of inactivity easily," says Dr. Hill.

For those folks who are completely inactive, though, there is good news. "You'll have the most to gain, even with just a small change," says Dr. Hill. "Research clearly shows that going from doing almost nothing to doing just a little holds the most potential for improvement in terms of overall health and maybe in terms of weight loss as well."

Your first step, then, is to aim low—reduce the nonactivity by at least 30 minutes. Then over time, keep chipping away. "By replacing 30 minutes of nothing with 30 minutes of some mild activity, you can burn off an extra 40 to 50 calories or more," says Dr. Hill. Decrease nonactivity by 60 minutes, and you'll burn off 100 or more calories, and so on. "The point isn't to replace that inactive time with high-impact aerobics but simply to get moving, even if it's a relaxing walk," says Dr. Hill.

If you're sedentary for five hours a day, you aren't off the hook. "It still couldn't hurt to knock 30 minutes to an hour off those five hours of inactivity," says Dr. Hill. Of course, if your job requires you to stay seated for that amount of time, you may have to create your calorie deficit elsewhere.

If you're only sedentary three hours a day, you may already lead an active daily life. Create your calorie deficit with either more daily activity (described in the next section) or planned exercise (discussed below).

Part II: Add On to Your Everyday Activities

Getting things done is its own kind of exercise and, like a robust workout, it burns calories. "Chores, office work, running errands— you can enlist all of them in achieving your weight-loss goal," says Dr. Hill. First, estimate how much time you spend being active during the day by answering the following questions.

1. How many hours on the job do you spend on your feet and moving throughout the day?
2. About how many flights of stairs do you climb during the day?
3. On average, how many miles do you walk a day (not including planned exercise, but the walking you do to and from work, in the hallways, running errands)?
4. On average, how many hours do you spend engaging in activities like gardening, chores and housecleaning during the day?

These questions can give you a good idea of how active you are above and beyond planned exercise. If you walk very little during the

day (less than a mile) but engage in one or two hours of strenuous chores, chances are you may already be doing pretty well in this department. If so, move to the planned-exercise section. But if you find that you're doing very little of any of the activities mentioned above, then this may be the right spot for running up a calorie deficit.

Look over the list of daily activities that follows and try to integrate them into your day. Some are simple little changes, others require a little more effort.

1. Instead of taking the elevator, take the stairs. The one to two minutes it takes to make it up a couple of flights can burn off 10 to 20 calories. "Two or three trips a day up the stairs—it adds up," says Dr. Hill.

2. Instead of spending your whole lunch break sitting and eating, take a one-mile walk before you eat. A stroll can burn off about 100 calories and may diminish appetite. Five days a week, that can add up to a sizable loss in pounds.

3. If you don't have time for a sustained walk, take brisk mini-walks of 5 to 10 minutes throughout the day. Thirty minutes total each day may burn an extra 150 calories.

4. Pick one part of the house or property that needs spot cleaning— whether it's window cleaning or mopping or scrubbing floors. Your residence may already be spotless, but consider the rewards: Scrubbing, mopping and window cleaning without pause can rack up 250 calories in one hour. Washing dishes can clear off 135 calories per hour, for example.

5. Do more standing. Standing for an hour amounts to only a 10- to 20-calorie difference over sitting for an hour, but it can add up. Deep in thought? Pace—for every 15 steps or so you'll burn a calorie.

6. Instead of using the company parking lot, park a few blocks away and walk. If you walk only one-fifth of a mile, that can burn off 20 to 25 calories. To and from work can deflate your day by 50 calories—250 calories for the week, weather permitting.

7. Get down to some serious lawn work: Rake the lawn, sack leaves,

cultivate a garden. Pushing a lawn mower burns 350 calories per hour; raking the lawn, 220 calories per hour; garden work, 250 calories per hour.

8. If you're at work and need to reach someone across the building, don't call—stop by her office instead. Reduce your phone calls and substitute person-to-person contact.

WORKOUTS—TAKE YOUR PICK

Which of the following activities sound appealing—and which leave you cold? Rate them from one to ten.

Mild to Moderate Exercise*	Calories Burned per Hour
Tennis	425
Bicycling or stationary cycling, 10 mph	415
Hiking with a 20-pound backpack, 3 mph	400
Aerobic exercise (moderate intensity)	350
Horseback riding	350
Roller skating	350
Square dancing	350
Treadmill walking, 4 mph	345
Ballroom dancing	300
Calisthenics	300
Rowing machine (easy)	300
Strength training	300
Table tennis	300
Aerobic exercise (low impact)	275
Golf, walking with clubs	270
Walking, (mild) 2 to 2.5 mph	185 to 255
Bicycling or stationary cycling, (slow) 5.5 mph	245

Now come up with a few activities of your own. Think about how you spend your day, and jot down some activities you could add to your daily schedule that would increase the amount of overall motion and help run up a calorie deficit. Remember—we aren't talking exercise. (That comes next.) We're talking simple movement. Then try them out.

Moderate to Intense Exercise*	Calories Burned per Hour
Martial arts	790
Running, 7.2 mph	700
Stair-climbing machine	680
Jumping rope	660
Bicycling or stationary cycling, 13 mph	655
Rowing machine (higher intensity)	655
Run/jog, 5.5 mph	655
Bench-stepping class (moderate intensity)	610
Cross-country skiing, 5 mph	600
Handball	600
Walking, (vigorous) 5 mph	555
Polka dancing	540
Swimming	540

*The caloric listings for all of the activities above are estimates based on what a 150-pound person might burn over one hour's time.

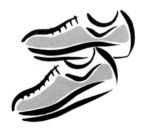

Part III: Start a Workout Routine You Can Live With

Your job keeps you on your toes, and you rarely find yourself sacked out in front of the tube. You also engage in lots of daily activities—schlepping groceries, walking to and from work, tending to your garden. In short, you are one busy woman. The best place to target your calorie deficit, then, may be in your planned exercise.

If you aren't getting at least three hours of aerobic exercise per week, consider upping the ante.

"Workouts—Take Your Pick" on page 182 is a list of activities, along with the number of calories they burn off by the hour. "The point isn't to choose an exercise according to how many calories it burns, but one which you enjoy most," says Dr. Hill. "The key to exercising regularly is whether you like the activity. Choose the one that grabs your fancy."

If your goal is to knock off 150, 300 or 450 calories each day, you can choose one activity to hit the deficit. Or treat it buffet-style: Burn some calories from one activity and some from another. The activities are grouped by intensity—mild to moderate, and moderate to intense. If you're an experienced exerciser, you can choose from the moderate- or high-intensity calorie burners. If you're just starting out, stick with the mild stuff—and enjoy yourself.

Dr. Hill offers this technique to help you make the right pick. Rate the activities from one to ten, based on how much you like them and how realistic it is for you to fit them into your day. "That helps you visualize the best choices—what really might work out for you and if you'll stick to it," says Dr. Hill.

A Beginner's Guide to Getting Fit

Step one: Consider the benefits of exercise. Step two: Pout if you must. Step three: Get motivated!

The very thought of going from zero fitness and marshmallow softness to full stamina, firmness and energy can seem overwhelming—enough to make you want to lie down. But you shouldn't think of getting into a regular exercise routine as a matter of suddenly beginning to exercise. Beginning an exercise program comes in stages, in tiny steps, many of which happen before you even slip on those walking shoes or enter the fitness center. The very fact that you're reading this chapter means that you're already in one of the important first stages. And continuing to exercise regularly is also a process of change, a cycle of smooth sailing and bumpy seas.

Fortunately, there are techniques that you can use to help you move to the next level. But first, take the quiz on page 186 to see where you are right now. Just be aware that the stage you are at changes all the time.

How to Keep Moving

Of course, once you know where you are, it's easy to see what's next. Here's how to get there.

Stage 1: I Don't Want to Exercise. If you are at this stage, you may be wondering what could possibly be done to get you to budge beyond it. Other people might be pressuring you, but it's up to you—you're the one who has to tie on your shoes and go out for a walk. And you don't even want to make the effort to think about it.

Two things can offer a nudge: Gathering Information and Ranting and Whining.

Gathering Information involves being open to facts and opinions concerning your state of fitness (or lack thereof) and both the benefits

ARE YOU WORKOUT-READY?

*F*igure out where you stand (or sit) by checking either True or False for the following questions.

True   **False**

☐   ☐   1. I don't want to exercise.

☐   ☐   2. I have thought about exercising, but no particular type appeals to me.

☐   ☐   3. I have thought about exercising, but I haven't made any plans to do so yet.

☐   ☐   4. I have thought about exercising, but I haven't actually tried it yet.

☐   ☐   5. I have thought about exercising and plan to try in the next month.

☐   ☐   6. I have thought about exercising and tried within the past year, but gave up.

☐   ☐   7. I have thought about exercising and have tried it in small bits.

☐   ☐   8. I have actually chosen some type of exercise.

☐   ☐   9. I have actually started working out regularly.

☐   ☐   10. I do work out fairly regularly.

Look at your check marks. Chances are, there were one or more questions you answered "True" to, and then all your answers after that were "False" (unless you happened to answer "True" to question ten). The number of the last question to which you answered "True" is your score.

If your score is . . .

1: You're in the "I Don't Want to Exercise" stage.

Between 2 and 5: You're in the "I'll Think about It" stage.

6 or 7: You're in the "I'm Almost Ready" stage.

8 or 9: You're in the "I'm Ready" stage.

10: You're in the "I'm Keeping On" stage.

of exercise and the health risks of not exercising. The source of the information can be external—others observing that you don't exercise, loved ones confronting you about it, family members giving you newspaper or magazine articles about exercise. Or it can be internal—watching TV programs or movies about sports, reading about exercise, learning about the psychology of why people don't exercise. In some cases, simply soaking up the incoming information can at least make you more likely to start thinking seriously about exercise, even if you have no intention (yet) of doing anything about it.

It could be, however, that despite the good efforts of your friends and relatives, the fact still remains that you don't want to exercise. And right now you simply may not be interested in gathering information.

So maybe you need to try Ranting and Whining. This involves giving vent to the problem. You may complain about what happened the last time you tried to exercise ("Oh, that cramp I got! I was sore for days!") or all the things that kept you from working out. All this talking and complaining about the problem at least gets you thinking about exercising. It gets the wheels turning so that getting fit becomes a problem to be solved.

It may seem that nothing is happening in the I-Don't-Want-to-Exercise stage, but the more you gather information and rant and whine, the more their effects can accumulate.

Stage 2: I'll Think about It. When you've reached this stage, not only are you more aware that a problem exists, you're also seriously considering doing something about it. This is great progress, even if you haven't actually made a commitment to start.

In this stage, you're considering the pros and cons of starting. You're at the point where you might increase your physical activity or decide you're not quite ready for prime-time—or any other time—workouts and give it up for now.

In this stage, you know where you want to go and you may even know how to get there. But you can't quite cajole yourself into following through with any action. Gathering Information and Ranting and Whining can be helpful here, as well as two other techniques: Role Modeling and Reinventing Yourself.

Role Modeling takes Gathering Information one step further. Here you closely observe someone you know, someone in the public eye or even some fictional character who might inspire you to fitness. You might chat with a friend who exercises regularly, or watch sporting events like the Olympics or movies with sports themes, like *Chariots of Fire* or *Hoosiers*. Who would be role models you respect and like? Pick some activity you might enjoy and watch a master of it. Once you open yourself up to the possibilities, you may be inspired to get moving yourself.

Reinventing Yourself involves looking at yourself in a different way.

Have you ever clutched a hairbrush in front of your dresser mirror, pretending to be a famous singer? This kind of fantasy is common in our teens and twenties but dies out as we get older. No matter what your age, now is the time to return to the power of fantasy. Try imagining yourself as an athlete or a dancer, or just someone who is really in shape.

Imagery could involve mentally picturing yourself as more flexible or thinner or whatever else exercise could help you with. Take three minutes, sit down, lean back, close your eyes and fantasize about downhill skiing, swimming, dancing or anything else physical that you want to try. Just do it.

When it's over, how does it feel? If you imagined skiing, could you feel the wind? The crouch? Did you see the hill, sun, snow, trees, other skiers? Could you feel the thrill in the pit of your stomach and

your head when the run was through? Make it happen in your mind.

You can also use imagery to conjure up a picture of yourself benefiting from exercise. Think of the thing exercise could help you with that is most important to you. Could your joints be more flexible? Would you be happier ten pounds lighter? Close your eyes. Imagine yourself moving as you would like to move. Watch this in the theater of your mind for however long it interests you. When you grow bored, stop, whether five seconds have passed or ten minutes. Repeat this two or three times a day.

It's even possible that performing certain movements in your mind rehearses the motor pathways so that when you do try the actual movement, it'll be easier.

Stage 3: I'm Almost Ready. This stage combines intending to change with making some small changes in behavior. In Stage 3, your intention and behavior crank up a notch. This means more Reinventing Yourself and imagery, plus some baby steps toward the real thing.

For example, exercising has been on Randy W.'s to-do list for years. After watching some aerobic and toning shows on TV, she fantasized about looking like the women on them. Then she decided she could do those exercises. She started making tapes of the shows so she could fit them in when her schedule permitted. Plus, she is walking to work more frequently now—she used to take a cab.

Stage 4: I'm Ready. Most people equate starting to exercise on a regular basis with change, overlooking the other steps that are part of the process. This is understandable, since in this fourth stage you actually choose some type of exercise or group of activities and start working out. People can see that you've changed your behavior in order to overcome the barriers or problems that have kept you from getting fit.

This is the riskiest stage. Many people overdo it. Then if they hurt or exhaust themselves, they become discouraged and drop back to I Don't Want to Exercise. If you have begun exercising and have kept at it for anywhere from one day to six months, you may think you're home free. Unfortunately, it's not so. For true change, you must also develop skills to keep from falling back and to deal with new problems.

One way to start is to announce to the world what you're about to undertake. Once you've publicly connected yourself with exercise, social support pushes you to keep the connection. If you stop, people may ask what happened, and you probably won't feel good about admitting failure.

Your pronouncement is your debut, your Coming Out. Coming Out is an important technique that is most useful in moving from preparation to action. You're declaring that the rest of your life will be different from your past. Your Coming Out could be as simple as buying your first pair of athletic shoes or joining a gym.

Stage 4 also involves making slight adjustments in your world. Move your exercise equipment to a more convenient location or join a gym that is on your way to or from work, or close enough to visit on your lunch hour, rather than one you have to make an effort to get to.

In this phase, you should give yourself plenty of positive reinforcement. Call a friend you haven't talked to in a while, or get tickets to a show or concert you would like to see. Use your imagination to reward yourself for signs of progress.

Stage 5: I'm Keeping On. Mastering this stage is crucial if exercising is to be an integral part of the rest of your life. The techniques for Keeping On are the sum of all the techniques that got you this far. So whatever tricks work for you, use them. It doesn't matter if they're different from the ones that help your best friend or that work for Cindy Crawford.

Remember what we said earlier: The stages of change are cyclical. You may work yourself all the way up to Keeping On, but then you get sick or injured, or take a trip or otherwise get distracted. You may even drop all the way back to I'm Thinking about It or even I Don't Want to Exercise. Nothing magical about reaching Keeping On will keep you there. If you find yourself at some lower level, you have to use the techniques appropriate to that level to climb back up. Then you may have to use bits of them to keep on Keeping On.

Caution: If you've made it to adulthood without exercising regularly or you haven't exercised in a while, be sure to talk with your physician. Let her know you plan to engage in mild to moderate aerobic exercise.

Yoga: The Gentlest Way to Shape Up

In the 1980s, we felt the burn. Now, burned out on high-impact fitness, many women have turned to the fluid postures of yoga.

*C*all it the yin and yang of fitness. The workout craze has been good for us, to be sure, but it has also exacted a cost. We've stepped, funked, jogged, in-line skated and pumped our bodies into shape. A backlash—or, to put it in a more karmic sense, a balance of energies—was inevitable.

As if on cue, the ancient Indian discipline of yoga has recently emerged as one of the hottest—and most tranquil—workouts. Yoga is turning up in health clubs, at one-on-one sessions with trainers, in the growing number of yoga studios and ashrams and on televisions all over the country. You gotta figure if Jane Fonda is making yoga videos, it's hot; her *Yoga Exercise Workout* video was the top seller for months.

Why the growing popularity? Because yoga provides an excellent combination of strength training and flexibility. It aligns the spine and improves circulation. It offers a unique way to sculpt long, lean— rather than bulked-up—muscles.

Yet some women aren't willing to give up the aerobic component to their fitness regimen altogether. And that's where the new brand of yoga comes in. A growing cadre of instructors is revamping the classic postures by picking up the pace and speeding sequences of poses to near-aerobic levels. Some of the newcomers even round out yoga classes with moves from other disciplines like kung fu and calisthenics. The result is a great workout that maintains all the stress-relieving qualities of the ancient discipline.

This yoga workout offers yet another way to shape up without strain. Only this approach, designed by New York City-based teacher and yoga therapist Allan Bateman, is about efficiency rather than speed. All yoga poses are performed slowly and mindfully, and there are pauses between postures as you recoup your energy.

But Bateman has no-nonsense Western instincts: He's extracted the essence of the poses and adapted them for our fast-moving culture. For instance, the warm-up doesn't begin, as most yoga sessions do, with a full-fledged Sun Salutation. Instead he gives us a streamlined version, pared down to the essential forward bend. Then he follows with a few basic maneuvers from *qi gong*, pronounced chee-GUNG (the Chinese energy-flow system that is the basis of tai chi), designed to teach the body subtle focus and control. Next he has us launch into a series of splits—lunges that strengthen the lower back and pelvic muscles while stretching the legs.

Then come two more postures—simplified versions of a traditional, complex series of movements—from the repertoire of poses taught at his Bateman Institute for Health Education.

Bateman recommends that these workouts be performed at least twice a week. As you grow more proficient, they'll become more challenging. At the end of your workout, you'll feel invigorated but calm—it's that yin and yang at work again.

Sun Stretch

An abbreviated version of the Sun Salutation, this stretch (see illustration on the opposite page) stimulates the circulation; tones the calves, hamstrings, buttocks and shoulders and stretches the spinal column.

1. Stand with your feet hip width apart. Clasping your thumbs, keep your arms straight and reach toward the ceiling, until your arms are beside your ears. When your back feels elongated and gently stretched, slowly lower your arms straight down, leading with your elbows, until your hands are dangling in front of your thighs.

2. Next, tuck your chin toward your chest and let your chin follow an imaginary line running down the center of your body toward the floor. You'll have a sense of unwinding, one vertebra at a time, from the base of the skull to the coccyx. Keep your knees straight but not locked.

3. When you've rounded over as far as is comfortable, cross your arms gently. Now just hang, letting gravity take over. Make sure

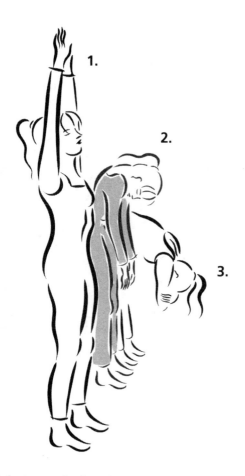

your weight is evenly distributed between the balls of your feet and your heels. Inhale slowly, through the nose, to a count of three. Exhale three counts through your nose. To come back up, let your arms go limp. Pull your navel in toward the tailbone and roll back up to a standing position. You should have a sense of your navel lifting each vertebra up to the base of the skull. Perform this move three times, allowing your movements to flow.

Qi Gong Relaxer

Not found in traditional yoga, this stretch subtly enhances energy awareness even as it relaxes the nervous system, slows the heart rate and lowers blood pressure.

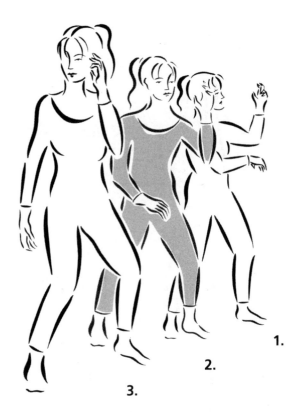

1.

2.

3.

1. Start with your feet shoulder width apart, knees slightly bent, back straight, hands resting on your thighs. Distribute your weight evenly between the balls of your feet and your heels. Raise your left arm, elbow slightly bent, so your left hand is in front of your left shoulder, palm facing right.

2. Slowly, as if you were pushing a cloud out of your way, push your arm across your body toward the right. At the same time, let your torso twist slightly to the right, so your shoulder moves with your arm. Your head and eyes should follow your hand.

3. When your left hand passes your right shoulder, let it float down. At the same time, begin the gesture with your right hand. Continue, alternating sides, and do six reps on each side. Keep your breathing gentle and the motion fluid.

Split

A streamlined version of the Warrior pose that develops pelvic and lower back muscles and increases range of motion on the inside, outside and backs of legs.

1. Stand with your legs as wide apart as is comfortable, toes pointing forward. Bend forward from your hips—think of them as a hinge—rather than from your waist. Allow your upper body to completely relax. Succumb to gravity. Cross your arms (gently, don't hold tight). Let them hang toward the floor. If you're very flexible, place your forearms on the floor. (Your hands or arms on the floor are there just to help you balance—let all the support come from your legs.) Lean back so your weight is over your heels. You'll feel the stretch up the backs of your legs. Hold for as long as is comfortable. Then place your palms on the floor, arms

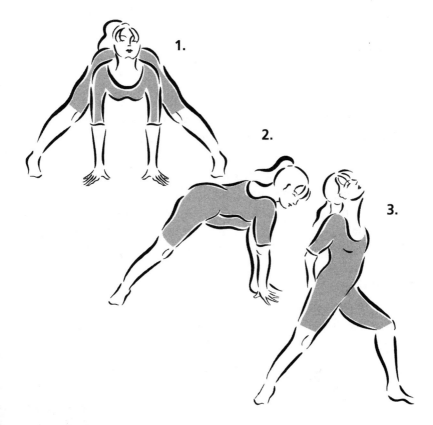

extended. Your chin should be lifted. Your back is parallel to the floor. Hold for as long as is comfortable.

2. Turn your left foot out 90 degrees. Swing your body over that knee so your chest is over your left thigh. Bend your left knee so that it's aligned directly between your ankle and toes; your right leg is straight behind you. Arms are extended on either side of your leg with fingertips touching the floor. Hold for as long as is comfortable.

3. Clasp your hands behind your back. Fingers are laced, palms facing behind you. Then lift your chin, head and shoulders upward, letting your back slowly arch. Direct your gaze to the ceiling. Your goal is to position your head directly above the hips and hold that position for ten seconds. This will take practice. The key here is to find your balance. To release, lower back down over your left thigh. Swing around to the center. Repeat three times on each side, alternating sides.

Jumps

Variations on the yoga split. These are incredible saddlebag busters that tone and strengthen all the muscles from the waist down.

1. Stand with your legs apart and your feet turned out, as shown in illustration on opposite page. Cross your arms at chest level and bend your knees.

2. Take an easy jump just a few inches off the floor. (If you have knee problems, you should use a mat.)

3. At the top of the jump, prepare for your landing on your toes and balls of your feet first, then your heels. The jumps should be one continuous, slow and fluid motion. Do three sets of six.

Cobra

A unique variant of the classic pose that keeps the vertebrae beautifully aligned and builds strength in the hamstrings, buttocks, back, chest, neck—and the eye muscles, too (see illustration on page 198).

1. Lie on your stomach, feet together, hands at your sides, palms up. Start by slowly directing your gaze in front of you, up the wall and

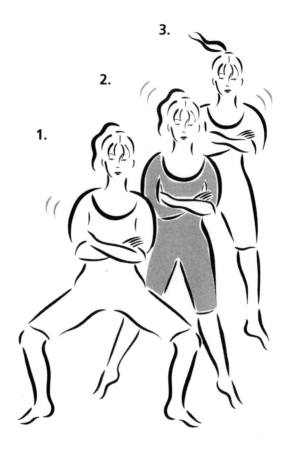

toward the ceiling. Then follow with your chin, using your back muscles to curl up.

2. When you can't go any farther, turn your palms over and slide your hands forward, lifting your chest off the floor. When your forearms are on the floor in front of you, hold for ten seconds.

3. Don't allow your navel to leave the floor, but—here's the challenge—bend your neck backward and try to look over your head toward your feet. *Stretch as far as you comfortably can*, without tensing your buttocks or straining your neck. If you can, slide your hands farther forward, extending your arms as far as possible while still keeping your navel on the floor. Don't shrug your shoulders. To come out of the Cobra, bend your elbows outward

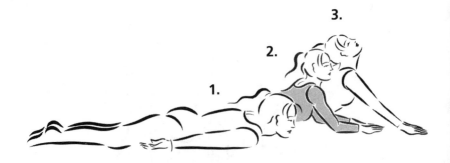

as you lower your body. Slide your arms back to your sides. Let your shoulders, chin and nose touch the floor. Repeat twice, allowing ten seconds to rise, ten seconds at the height of the pose and ten seconds to lower.

Do the Stroll

Want to lose weight, gain energy and live longer?
Put on your walking shoes and hit the road!

You lead a very busy life. You run a lot of errands—in your car. And you love to play games—like Pictionary. If this sounds like you, believe it or not you're sedentary. And folks who don't exercise just don't live as long as folks who do.

The good news is that you don't have to join a gym or buy a bike to become more fit. You can significantly improve your health—and keep your mind and body young—simply by **doing** something you learned as a kid: walking.

Come On, Step Right Up

Here's how walking regularly can benefit your health.

It trims you down. As you'd expect, walking tones your leg muscles so that they appear slimmer and more muscular. And it's no surprise that walking also helps promote long-term weight loss. But the benefits of pounding the pavement go far beyond a reduced girth and great gams. A study done at the University of California at Berkeley found a striking loss of fat from the *arms* of walkers after six months of regular exercise. In fact, walking can send fat fleeing from *all* parts of your body, says Grant Gwinup, M.D., the study's chief researcher.

It peps you up. In addition to trimming and toning your body, walking shapes up your insides. It benefits your circulatory system directly by strengthening your heart and enhancing the flow of oxygen to your brain. And a brain full of oxygenated blood means higher spirits and extra get-up-and-go.

Walking also gives your lungs a workout, which makes your breathing and metabolism more efficient. As a result, your overall stamina and endurance will increase, and you'll feel more energized all day long. In addition, you'll feel better about yourself with every step you take because you'll feel and look better, too.

Hitting the high road even improves your mental abilities. Researchers at Scripps College in Claremont, California, discovered that, in a group of adults between the ages of 55 and 91, those who exercised performed significantly better on all reasoning tests, all reaction-time tests and most memory tests.

It reduces your risk. If you have a sedentary lifestyle, a walking program can be your best health insurance policy—a policy to *prevent* disease, not pay for its treatment. (You can count yourself among the sedentary if the longest amount of time you spend in continuous full-body movement is less than 15 minutes twice a week.)

In addition to helping you reap the health benefits of avoiding weight gain, walking can do a lot to bring down mildly high blood pressure. Because walking prompts blood vessels to dilate, your blood can flow through them more easily, which causes your pressure to drop. Also, walking helps reduce stress—a definite plus when high blood pressure is a problem.

What's more, walking helps to lower your total blood-cholesterol level while raising the level of high-density lipoprotein (HDL) cholesterol (the kind that helps keep your arteries from getting clogged).

For all of these reasons, strolling goes a long way toward reducing your risk of developing heart disease.

It lengthens your life span. In an ongoing study of the health and lifestyles of 16,936 Harvard alumni, researchers found that in all age groups, death rates decreased as physical activity increased. The men who burned 2,000 or more calories per week through exercise had a 28 percent lower death rate than men who exercised less or not at all. The bottom line: Walk regularly, and you can strut your stuff for many more years. Think of it this way: "For every hour you walk, you can add an hour to your life," says Ralph Paffenbarger, Jr., M.D., Ph.D., one of the study's authors.

Ready, Set, Walk!

Want to start logging some life-lengthening miles? It's as easy as it sounds. Just follow this simple ten-step plan, and you'll be strolling down the road to better health.

Get approval. If you haven't exercised in a while or have never walked for exercise, see your doctor for a checkup and tell her of your plans to begin a walking program.

Draft a contract. To help you focus on your goal—and then stick with it—write up a document that states what you want to accomplish. Include when, where, how long and how often you'll walk. As you reach your goals, reward yourself with a healthful treat such as a new pair of walking shoes.

Choose good shoes. Walking may be the cheapest form of transportation, but it's not free. To avoid injury and enhance enjoyment, you'll need to invest in a good pair of walking shoes. While almost any type of athletic shoes will work, you may want to try ones made specifically for walking.

Warm up. Stretching your muscles before walking will decrease your risk of injuring them. Then get your legs and body primed for action by walking slowly for a few minutes.

Take it slow. At first, try walking for 5 to 10 minutes. Do this every day for a week to get your muscles and feet accustomed to the exercise. During the second week of your walking program, take several 5- to 10-minute walks throughout the day. (This is less likely to

HOW FAST? HOW HARD?

You might think you'll have to chug along as fast as your feet will carry you to reap the benefits of walking. Not so, say the experts.

In a recent study, women who walked leisurely 20-minute miles recorded the same 6 percent increase in high-density lipoprotein (HDL) cholesterol (the good kind) as women who power-walked 12-minute miles. That jump in HDL translates to an 18 percent drop in heart disease risk.

What really counts when walking is how long you walk, not how fast you go. Just be sure you're not pushing too hard. "You should be able to talk while you walk," says Jerome Brandon, Ph.D., an exercise physiologist at Georgia State University in Atlanta. If you can't chat about the weather while you're walking, shift it down a gear—but if you can sing opera arias, it's time to pick up the pace a bit.

leave you with sore muscles or blisters than if you take one long walk.) Each week after that, gradually increase the amount of time you walk until you're walking at least 30 to 40 minutes total per day, no fewer than three times a week.

Perfect your posture. When you walk, stand tall, relax your shoulders and let your arms swing naturally. Keep your pelvis tucked forward so your lower back remains as straight as possible.

Chart your course. When you begin your program, walk at the same time and in the same place every day, if possible. This will help get you into the habit of walking. After a few weeks, you can vary your route. If you're walking along streets that don't have sidewalks, be sure to walk facing oncoming traffic. If you're walking at night, carry a flashlight and wear light-colored or reflective clothing.

Cool down. At the end of your trek, slow your pace and wind down. Then follow the same stretching routine you used for warming up.

Keep an exercise journal. To track your progress, write down how far and how long you walked each day. You can also add inspiring quotes or jot down what you saw or how you felt while walking.

Listen to your body. When you first begin your walking program, you may experience some fatigue or find that you're breathing harder or that your heart's pumping faster than usual. These changes simply mean that your body is adjusting to your new exercise routine. However, if you experience any pain, stop exercising and see your doctor. Above all, walking should be pain-free and fun.

Tone Up While You Trim Down

Resistance training can firm and tone your body without turning you into the Incredible Hulk-ette.

For many women, middle age most notably hits right around the middle. But packing on additional pounds is only half the problem: Even if your scale hasn't budged much over the years, what was once muscle may have been replaced by fat. And fat around the abdominal organs is believed to balloon the risk of heart disease, diabetes and certain kinds of cancer.

But don't despair. You can get your 25-year-old body back at any age. What it takes is a regimen that includes 1) vigilantly adhering to a healthy, low-fat, low-calorie, high-fiber diet; 2) dedicating at least 45 minutes a day to fitness walking or some other moderately vigorous aerobic activity; and, perhaps most important, 3) embracing a program of resistance training.

Research suggests that dusting off the dumbbells (and using them) may replace fat with muscle. In this study, 13 men around age 60 got rid of about four pounds of fat and built about four pounds of muscle while following an average four-month-long resistance-training program.

The guys liked their tighter look and extra energy. But the researchers were impressed by the fact that almost half of the fat the men lost was that potentially dangerous central-body fat. Just published research suggests that resistance training could give older women the same good deal.

"Older people have more to gain by beginning a resistance training program," says study author Ben F. Hurley, Ph.D., director of the exercise science lab at the University of Maryland in College Park. "Younger people have a greater reserve of muscle and strength. But as we age, strength training becomes more important because many older people become sedentary and start to lose valuable muscle."

While aerobic workouts are still the most efficient way to burn calories and reduce your fat stores, resistance training is the key to building up your active muscle tissue for long-lasting increases in metabolism. The more muscle you have, the quicker your metabolism and the easier it is to keep pounds and inches at bay.

Age is no barrier to stoking your body's calorie-burning furnace, either. In fact, a recent study found that elderly people in a resistance-training program required about 15 percent more calories than they needed during their sedentary days just to maintain their weight.

Get Your Twentysomething Body Back

Want to get back where you belong—perhaps even look better than you did at 25? *Prevention* magazine asked Daniel Kosich, Ph.D., senior consultant to IDEA: International Association of Fitness Professionals, to design a resistance workout to complement a healthy diet and aerobics routine and help you look toned, trimmed and proportioned. We also requested that the workout be easy to follow whether or not someone belongs to a gym.

Some of these exercises are most effective when done with dumbbells. If you haven't been working out with weights, first try the exercises without any. Then add a 1- or 2-pound set of dumbbells and gradually work your way up to 5, 10 or 15 pounds for some of the exercises.

To squeeze the most from your efforts, Dr. Kosich advocates using the principle of progressive resistance: Work each muscle to the max by doing each exercise until you can't do any more while still maintaining good form. Build up to the maximum number of repetitions and sets given next to each exercise, then move up to the next heavier weight and build up from the beginning again. Keep all the exercises slow and controlled, and rest about one minute between sets. Do this workout two to three times a week.

Easy-Does-It Push-Ups

An excellent workout for your chest, shoulders and the backs of your arms, push-ups don't require weights and can be modified for most anyone. If you're really out of shape or have bad knees, start by doing them against the wall. Facing the wall, stand about arm's length away and place your palms on the wall. Now, bend your elbows, lower yourself toward the wall and then push yourself back to starting position. Don't worry if your heels come off the floor a bit.

To do regular push-ups, start with your knees on the ground. Place your hands on the floor slightly wider than shoulder width apart. Be careful not to arch your back. Holding your tummy in helps. Keep your eyes to the ground to maintain your neck in a neutral position. Do as many push-ups as you can in this position, working up to two sets of 25. When you've mastered these, you may want to switch to a straight-legged (toes and hands on the floor) position for an added challenge.

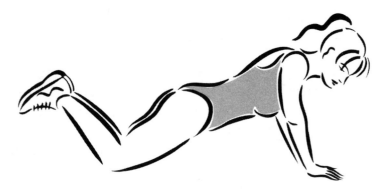

Pull-Ups Anyone Can Do

Pull-ups work the biceps and the latissimus dorsi, the long muscles that line the sides of your back and create an attractive V-shaped body when toned. You'll need a bar or a portable bar that adjusts to fit the doorways in your home. (These are available in most sporting-goods stores.) Keep your hands slightly wider than your shoulders. Do these with palms facing you for an effective biceps workout. Beginners should put a chair beneath and to the side of the bar to boost themselves into the starting position. Begin in the up position. Now lower yourself until your elbows are just slightly bent. Then, using the chair, boost yourself back to the starting position and repeat. As you become stronger, you'll be able to pull yourself back up without using the chair.

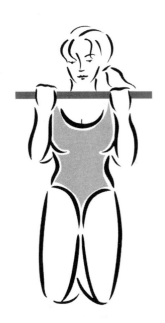

Pull-ups are difficult, so try not to get discouraged. Just do as many as you can, eventually working your way up to five or ten.

Crunches for the Tummy

Crunches are great for toning your abdominal muscles. To do them, lie on your back and keep your knees bent, feet flat on the floor. Lift your upper body until your shoulder blades are just off the floor, and then lower. Cross your hands over your chest or put them behind your head, but be careful not to pull against your head—let your abdominals do all the work. Hold your head in a neutral position (not crooked forward or back). You should be able to fit your fist between your throat and chin. Work up to two sets of 25.

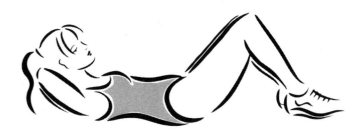

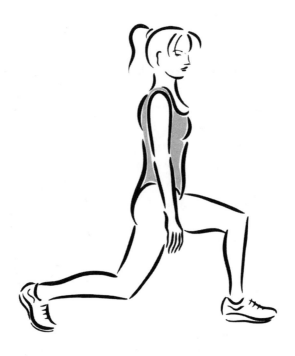

S-L-O-W Lunges

Lunges also work all the muscles of your legs and buttocks. Start with one foot in front of the other and lower your back knee toward the floor, then come back up. Keep your front knee aligned over your front foot to make sure you bend your knee no more than 90 degrees. Don't lean forward—your torso should drop like a plumb line. You can hold onto a chair for balance. Repeat with the other knee in front. Work up to three sets of 12.

When you are able to complete all three sets of regular lunges, progress to the more advanced step lunge. Start with your feet together, step forward with one foot, drop your back knee straight down toward the floor, then press up with your front leg and return to starting position. Repeat with the other leg stepping to the front. Keep the movement slow and controlled to prevent straining your knees. You can add a pair of dumbbells at your sides or resting on your shoulders, for more resistance.

Super Squats

Squats shape the fronts and backs of your thighs as well as your buttocks and calves. They are most effective when done with dumbbells held at your sides or resting on your shoulders. Stand with your feet slightly wider than your shoulders and slightly turned out. Begin with a partial squat, knees bent about 45 degrees. Do as many as you can, working up to three sets of 12. Progress to a 90-degree squat (knees bent at right angles, so you feel like you're lowering yourself into a chair). Keep your abs tucked in and your back straight.

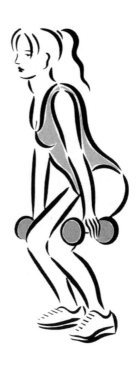

If you have a history of knee problems, check with your doctor to make sure you can do these and the following exercise without straining these joints.

Supine Flies for Beginners

These work the chest and the fronts of the shoulders. Lie with your back on a bench. Keep one or both feet on the bench to keep

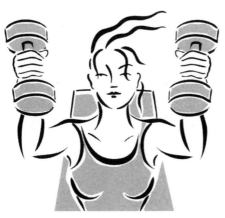

from arching your back. Start with light weights, extending your arms out to your sides (at right angles to your body) with elbows slightly bent. Pull the dumbbells straight over your chest, until they just about meet. Maintain the tension in your chest and shoulders to control the movement back down. Work up to one to three sets of 12.

Prone Reverse Flies: Do's and Don'ts

These work the upper back and rear shoulders. Lie on your chest on a bench, turning your head to the side. The weights should hang from your hands below the bench. Pull the weights straight out to your sides by squeezing your shoulder blades together. Do not jerk the weights up. Work up to one to three sets of 12.

Seated Lateral Raises: The Key Is Control

These strengthen and shape the shoulders. Sitting on a chair, hold weights at your sides. Lift the weights straight out to each side until your hands are at shoulder height, keeping a slight bend at the elbows. As you raise and lower the weights, palms face the floor. Work up to one to three sets of 12.

Arm and Leg Raises: The Final Touch

These strengthen the lower back. Lie with your stomach on the floor, arms overhead. Turn your head to one side.

Slowly lift your right arm and left leg straight up, and then over. Repeat, using your opposite arm and leg. This is a small movement. Press your hips and shoulders to the floor to keep from rotating. Work up to one to two sets of ten on each side.

PART SIX

Age-Defying Beauty Secrets

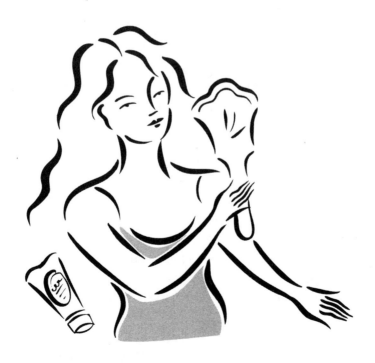

Young Skin for Life

When it comes to youthful-looking skin, the best offense is a good defense.

Ever look into your mirror and wonder what you're going to look like 10 years from now? Even 30? While there's no telling for sure when crow's-feet will strike, there's no reason not to be prepared. And while you can't stop the physical process of aging, you can slow the inevitable, or minimize it, through reasonable maintenance. Recent skin-care advances in everything from sun protection to wrinkle-fighting alpha hydroxy acids (AHAs) and even cosmetic surgery mean the outlook is much brighter than ever before. Here's what experts say about how your face changes through the years, what you can expect and how to cope.

The following tackles the skin's aging process decade by decade. The predictions that follow will vary depending on how dark or fair your skin is naturally. Melanin-rich skin is thicker than fair skin and more effectively resists signs of aging. Sun exposure matters, too: A woman who has fried her face every summer will age faster than one who has lived her entire life indoors. For the last word on what you should do, see your dermatologist.

The Twenties: Preserving Perfection

What to expect: Somewhat oily skin and, as a result, occasional acne. According to Andrew J. Scheman, M.D., assistant clinical professor at Northwestern University Medical School in Chicago and co-author of *The Cosmetics Buying Guide*: "After age 20, the amount of collagen (which helps keep skin plump and firm) decreases by about 1 percent per year. But it's a very gradual process." You won't notice wrinkles yet! Sun exposure ages your skin faster than anything else. You can control this. "The sun breaks down collagen and elastin," says Mary Ellen Brademas, M.D., associate clinical professor at New York University Medical Center in New York City. "Skin is not plumped up the way it used to be."

"Seventy-eight percent of sun damage is done before the age of 18," according to Arnold W. Klein, M.D., a Beverly Hills dermatologist and associate clinical professor at the University of California, Los Angeles, School of Medicine, who emphasizes establishing good patterns in your adolescence. "The skin has an ability to repair itself," he says, "but you shouldn't keep insulting it. The most important thing is to use sunscreens judiciously."

What you can use:
- Toners for oily skin (Shiseido Pureness Balancing Lotion Oil Control)
- Soaps and cleansers with benzoyl peroxide or salicylic acid for acne (Neutrogena Oil Free Acne Wash)
- Eye cream (Clarins Eye Contour Gel)
- Oil-free moisturizer only if you need it (Catherine Atzen A.M.-P.M. Moisturizing Gel)
- AHA products that help clear up acne (Erno Laszlo Beta Complex Acne Treatment)
- Broad-spectrum sunscreen with a sun protection factor (SPF) of at least 15 (Lancome Sunblock Face Creme AntiWrinkle SPF 25)

What a dermatologist might do: Treat acne and early signs of sun damage with glycolic acid peels (50 percent to 70 percent strength), Retin-A or, in extreme cases, Accutane.

The Thirties: Proper Care = Big Benefits

What to expect: "Aging really begins at 30," says Dr. Brademas. Your skin gets stiffer because you lose collagen and elastic fibers that are the underlying support structures. Skin also gets drier because of a slow decline in oil production. It thins because you lose fat pads and starts to sag from gravity's pull. Your skin also ages on the surface.

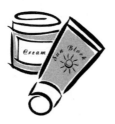

As your elastic fibers degenerate, the skin becomes less resilient, and so the pull of the muscles (when you smile, frown, squint) becomes etched into the skin. Even sleep affects the way we look. "The lines from the nose to the mouth will run deeper on the side you sleep on, and the corner of your mouth will be longer," says Dr. Klein. Of course, people age at an individual rate. As Dr. Brademas says, "It depends on genetics, how much smoking you've done and how much you've abused yourself with the sun."

You're likely to have normal (that is, "combination") skin that's oily in the T-zone; adult acne from stress, pregnancy, birth control pills or fertility drugs; early signs of crow's-feet, smile lines, forehead creases and frown lines (vertical lines between brows); and thinning lips. Early sun abuse may result in age spots (solar lentigines), acne rosacea (a blotchy, rashlike condition) and a sallower complexion.

What you can use:
- Gentle soap or cleanser (M.D. Formulation Facial Cleanser Basic)
- Toner for normal to dry skin (Mary Kay Gentle Action Freshener Formula I)
- Water-based moisturizer (Biotherm Biofluide Pure Oil-Free Hydrating Lotion)
- Eye cream (Loreal Plenitude Eye Defense Gel-Cream)
- Sunscreen (Garden Botanika Chemical-Free Sunblock SPF 15)
- AHAs and other exfoliants (Avon Anew Protecting Lotion for Problem Skin)

What a dermatologist might do: Treat sun damage with Retin-A and glycolic acid peels (50 percent to 70 percent) to minimize pores, soften fine lines and improve skin tone. (The anti-acne drug Accutane also shrinks pores, one reason many blemish-free women take it. But since it causes birth defects, "it's irresponsible to endorse Accutane for pore size," says one dermatologist who spoke anonymously.)

The Forties: Rescue Remedies That Work

What to expect: Normal skin with an increasingly dry T-zone. Crow's-feet, smile lines, deep smile lines from nose to mouth, forehead creases, frown lines, lines above the lips (even if you don't smoke), undereye bags, thinning lips and dilated pores on the nose (from oil glands that enlarge with age), sun damage in the form of sun or age spots and actinic keratoses (small, scaly sun-induced precancerous growths). "After 40 the skin doesn't rebound as quickly," says Dr. Klein, "so people should be very careful about weight loss and gain. Fat redistributes—it doesn't always go back to where it came from."

What you can use:
- Cleansing creams (Prescriptives All Clean Soothing Cream)
- Toner (Clinique Clarifying Lotion 2)
- AHAs and other exfoliants (Black Opal Skin Retexturizing Complex)
- Water-based moisturizer (Yves Saint Laurent Prevention+/Time Prevention Day Creme and Elizabeth Arden Ceramide Time Complex Capsules)
- Eye cream (Maybelline Revitalizing Opium Eye Treatment Cream)
- Sunscreen (Physicians Formula Sun Shield for Faces Formula SPF 20)

What a dermatologist might do: Treat sun damage with Retin-A or glycolic acid peels; acne or acne rosacea with Retin-A or Accutane; sun spots and actinic keratoses with liquid nitrogen or a laser. Use fillers (collagen, fat transplants, Fibrel) or mild trichloroacetic acid peels to smooth out lines and plump up lips; and Botox (a botulism toxin that in small amounts temporarily paralyzes tiny facial nerves) to relax deep frown lines on the forehead.

The Fifties: Know Your Options

What to expect: Drier skin. Adult acne that may flare up with menopause (but will usually subside afterward). "The loss of elastic fibers in the skin accelerates tremendously after age 50," says Dr. Scheman. The results: eyelid droop, undereye bags, marionette lines (from corners of mouth to chin). Gravity also takes its toll on cartilage, says Dr. Klein: The tip of the nose begins to fall down, the ears start to elongate and the jawline becomes less angular because of underlying bone loss. "This is the best decade for anti-aging facial surgery," says Robert Kotler, M.D., an otolaryngologist and clinical instructor of head and neck surgery at the University of California, Los Angeles, School of Medicine. The reason? "Most women are pretty healthy now, but in their sixties and seventies, they can develop a medical condition that precludes having a procedure."

Lastly, changing your appearance is less startling if you do it in your fifties. Says Dr. Kotler, "A woman who has all of these procedures done at age 60, who suddenly looks 40, well, it's a little too much sometimes." So the time to strike, if you must, is now.

What you can use:

- Oil-based soaps and cleansers (Le Teint Ricci Delicate Cleansing Bar)
- Alcohol-free toner (Nivea Visage Alcohol Free Moisturizing Facial Toner)
- Moisturizer (Institut Esthederm Intensive Cream 10% Collagen Nourishing Cream)
- AHAs and other exfoliants (La Prairie Age Management Intensified Serum)
- Eye cream (Alexandra de Markoff Fresh Eye Cream)
- Firming cream (DeCleor Super Lifting Excellence Face Firming Lotion)
- Sunscreen (Vaseline Intensive Care Block Out Moisturizing Sunblock Lotion SPF 40+)

What a dermatologist might do: Use fillers, trichloroacetic acid peels, as above, and suggest corrective measures.

What a facial surgeon might do:

- A mild phenol chemical skin peel, stronger than a trichloroacetic acid peel, to remove lines, age spots, even some scars
- Upper eyelid surgery (to remove the fold of skin that forms between eyelash and eyebrow that conceals the natural eyelid); lower eyelid surgery (to remove bags under eyes)
- Face- and neck-lift (to remove jowls and tighten brow, cheeks, jawline and neck)

The Sixties: Protect, Protect, Protect!

What to expect: All the problems of the fifties, plus jowls (caused by resorption of bone in the upper and lower jaw). "The lower third of the face collapses because as people get older they lose their facial skeleton," says Dr. Klein. "That's why people's chins fall down. And we lose dentition. People tend to forget that their teeth are helping to support the lower third of their face." So it's important to see a dentist regularly. Moreover, a woman might consider corrective measures at this juncture—stronger chemical and surgical techniques. Says Dr. Kotler, "A phenol peel continues to be the most important procedure because it removes wrinkles. You can undergo a high-quality face- and neck-lift, but if your skin still looks old, you look old."

What you can use:
- Soapless cleanser (Chanel Cleansing Milk)
- Alcohol-free toner (Almay Sensitive Care Toner)
- Oil-based day moisturizer and night cream (Pevonla Reactive Skin Care Cream and Princess Marcella Borghese Cura Notte/Night Therapy for Dry to Very Dry)
- AHAs and other exfoliants (Estee Lauder Fruition Triple ReActivating Complex)
- Firming cream, if desired (Sothy Vitality Serum)
- Eye cream (Ultima II Brighten Up, Tighten Up Eye Cream)
- Sunscreen (Bioelements Sun Diffusing Protector SPF 15)

What a dermatologist might do: Use fillers, trichloroacetic acid peels, as above, and suggest corrective measures.

What a facial surgeon might do:
- Upper and lower eyelid surgery
- An "aggressive" face- and neck-lift
- A medium or heavy-strength phyto peel

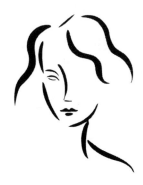

Environmental Protection for Your Complexion

Neither sun, nor pollution, nor a shrinking ozone layer need keep your skin from looking its best.

A diminishing ozone layer, humidity, dryness, pollution—what's a beleaguered complexion to do? Each of these environmental elements presents a different hazard for your skin, from premature aging and breaking out to dry, itchy skin and skin cancer. The good news is, your skin is a wonderfully adaptable organ, and with some help from our experts and some common sense, it can meet and defeat these challenges.

The First Deadly Skin Sin

There's little disagreement that the single most important environmental factor that affects skin is sunlight. "Sunlight is the major cause of skin cancer and skin aging," says Peyton E. Weary, M.D., professor of dermatology at the University of Virginia School of Medicine in Charlottesville and president of the American Academy of Dermatology.

To underscore this cause for concern about the sun's rays, there is now reliable evidence from a recent study done in Toronto, Canada, indicating that depletion of the ozone layer is allowing a greater amount of UVB sunlight (the shorter rays mainly responsible for burning) to penetrate to the surface of the earth.

"The theoretical concerns are very serious, and we need to take them seriously," says Dr. Weary. "For instance, we already know a lot about the relationship between sunlight and certain forms of skin cancer. But beyond that, I think that there's a lot of things we don't know about the connection between immune suppression and sunlight."

You should get into the habit of wearing a sunscreen every time you go out—like a second skin. But sunscreen use, while vital, is not enough. "We have to realize that the use of sunscreens should not encourage us to go out and spend long periods in the sun when we don't need to," says Dr. Weary. This doesn't mean you should shun the sun. In fact, it's fine to participate in outdoor activities. But when you do, you should use an effective sunscreen (sun protection factor 15 or higher), applied every two hours in proper amounts. (About one ounce is necessary to cover the body surface.)

"In addition," says Dr. Weary, "wear protective clothing, including a hat with a broad four-inch brim, and try to schedule outdoor activities to avoid the peak sun hours from about 10:00 A.M. to 3:00 P.M.

"We also feel strongly that people should stay out of tanning parlors," says Dr. Weary. There are over a million people going to tanning salons on a regular basis. "There's no question that tanning salons cause damage to the skin. They're causing it particularly because they use UVA (long-wavelength ultraviolet light). This UVA radiation is probably causing more aging changes than the shorter UVB wavelengths because it penetrates more deeply into the skin and therefore damages the collagen or connective tissue.

"So people who use tanning parlors regularly are likely to wind up with leathery, old-looking skin. There's no question about the fact that most of the major 'aging changes' are sun-induced," says Dr. Weary.

Hot Weather Hygiene

People who live in highly humid climates or spend long periods immersed in water face another environmental hazard for their skin. Fungus, yeast and bacterial infections are much more common in tropical climates: All the elements needed for them to flourish and grow more luxuriantly are present in moist, humid environments.

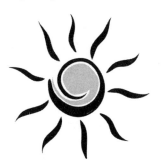

People who wear rubber-soled shoes in warm climates are also generally at still higher risk for infections on their feet because the rubber traps moisture. A good hygiene program and use of antibacterial soaps in areas where the skin overlaps can help prevent these problems.

"Powders are sometimes helpful in these moist areas where skin folds overlap," says Dr. Weary. "You have to be very careful when using them, however. You shouldn't let this stuff accumulate, because powders get to be kind of gritty after a while, and you can get 'pilling'—little balls of powder that can irritate the skin. These areas must be well-cleaned."

More Face-Saving Strategies

Whether we're trying to counteract the effects of air pollution, high humidity or almost any skin problem you can think of, good skin cleansing is a key player in the plan for healthy skin. Not only can it remove the grit of city pollution but it also helps to reduce the accumulation of dead skin cells and bacteria.

A word of caution, however—this does not necessarily mean scrubbing—and it never means scrubbing when we're talking about your face. Vigorous rubbing may feel like it's getting you really clean, but in fact it can do more harm than good.

Regular bathing and the use of mild soaps are great weapons in the battle for healthy skin. "I recommend that my patients stay away from a lot of the detergent soaps," says Dr. Weary. "They can be quite irritating to the skin and overdry it."

Milder soaps, such as those soaps that are glycerin-based or those that have lubricants in them, are particularly helpful for people who have to compensate for low humidity, outdoors or in the home. "Lack of proper humidity is a growing problem for people's complexions in today's climate-controlled environments such as air conditioning or forced-air heat," says Dr. Weary.

Moisturizers are the sunscreens of an air-conditioned environment—your best weapon. To prevent the dry, itchy skin associated with dehydrated environments, it's especially beneficial to use your moisturizer immediately after bathing while your skin is still slightly damp.

Blemish-Proof Your Complexion

While you're never too old to get a pimple, there's a right way and a wrong way to treat a breakout. These tips can help.

*B*lemishes don't discriminate by age, sex—or anything else. They happen to 15-year-olds before the prom and to 45-year-old executives before board meetings. But if they're only an occasional problem, you can help solve it yourself by using a simple prevention/treatment program.

Hands Off That Zit!

Your main goal should be to keep those frustrating, isolated blemishes—what dermatologists call grade-one acne—from turning into full-blown acne. Unfortunately, it's easy to take a simple, mild case of acne and make it into a messy condition by doing the wrong thing.

"The worst thing that most people do is to overscrub their skin," says Nelson Lee Novick, M.D., associate clinical professor of dermatology at Mount Sinai School of Medicine in New York City. "I recommend that my patients do not use washcloths or polyester scrub sponges. You should just wash gently with your fingertips and lightly pat dry with a soft towel when done. I don't like abrasive soaps or cleansers, either. They only irritate the whitehead. Instead, you should use a very mild soap—like one of those designed for sensitive skin. In short, there is no magic to cleansing—it's just removing surface dirt and oil—it won't make your acne disappear."

Whiteheads are underneath the surface of the skin but are embedded too deeply to be uprooted by cleansing. "If you vigorously scrub your skin to unseat them, you end up with the same number of blemishes, but you may rupture the whitehead below the surface, triggering the whole acne cascade," says Dr. Novick.

If you understand the chain reaction known as the acne cascade, you'll see why it's important to avoid it. "Think of the whitehead (made up of materials including oil-gland secretions, bacteria, fatty acids and dead skin cells) as a piece of TNT underneath your skin in the hair follicle. The detonator can be anything from nervous tension—good or bad—to physical stresses like rubbing," says Dr. Novick.

"Once the whitehead is triggered, the materials accumulate in it like water inside a closed balloon. The acne bacteria then have more material to break down into irritating fatty acids. Those fatty acids help to annoy and attack the remaining intact wall of the whitehead and eventually it ruptures, spewing its contents under the surface of your skin." This spillage, in turn, signals the body to attack the foreign material, causing an inflammatory reaction that may result in pimples, pustules, cysts and, eventually, scarring.

Another problem with overcleansing is that you can end up with extremely dry skin. This is a double whammy because acne medications—over-the-counter or prescription—tend to dry your skin. "Couple that with overzealous scrubbing and you can end up with skin that's like the Mojave Desert and far too sensitive to put any of the topical medications on," says Dr. Novick.

Other inappropriate measures include picking or squeezing the skin, which aggravates these blemishes below the surface. "The whitehead has nowhere to go unless the surface is opened mechanically, which I don't recommend people do for themselves," says Dr. Novick. "So it explodes below the surface, starting the acne cascade."

A common misconception is that the sun will have some beneficial effect on blemishes. In fact, the ultraviolet rays that penetrate the skin's surface can damage the follicles, closing them off and triggering an acne flare-up. Since it usually happens two to four weeks after sun exposure, people don't usually relate the breakout to the insult from the sun. Of course, wrinkles and skin cancer are also results of sun exposure.

What about Moisturizer?

Acne starts well below the surface. So drying out the surface—which is, unfortunately, what many acne medications do as a side

SKIN THAT "SQUEAKS" BREEDS BLEMISHES

Vigorous cleansing of your face can do much more harm than good. Resist the impulse to scrub skin until it's squeaky-clean and follow these simple steps to a clearer complexion.

1. Wash your hands. You wouldn't wash with a dirty washcloth.

2. Choose sensitive-skin bars or sensitive-skin liquid cleansers.

3. Moisten your face with lukewarm water to allow the cleanser to disperse more evenly.

4. Work your cleanser into a lather with your hands; this helps to save you from rubbing your face.

5. Gently wash your face, using just the pads of your fingertips to distribute the lather.

6. Rinse thoroughly by splashing your face with lukewarm water until the lather is completely gone.

7. Pat dry gently.

effect to their benefits (their antibiotic, unclogging actions)—is not necessarily a good thing. One way to counteract this side effect is to use a moisturizer.

"Use a moisturizer that's oil-free, hypoallergenic and fragrance-free," says Dr. Novick. "Some actually say nonacnegenic or noncomedogenic on their labels, which means that they won't promote blemishes. I usually recommend a simple formula—like a fragrance-free, hypoallergenic, noncomedogenic moisture lotion. The fewer ingredients, the less your skin has to react to. I'd suggest that you use your acne preparations at night and the moisturizer in the morning. The fact is, anything you put on your face should be simple."

Banish Blemishes with Benzoyl Peroxide

In an over-the-counter antiblemish product, you should choose one that has the one-two punch of an antibacterial and an unclogging effect.

"Look for something with 2.5 percent benzoyl peroxide, which is probably one of the most effective antiblemish medications," says Dr. Novick. "And look for a product that contains sulfur, sulfur and salicylic acid, or resorcinol, which are antibacterials and pore uncloggers."

When should you seek professional help? "If after two to four weeks of using an appropriate, mild, anti-acne regimen, cleansing properly and protecting from overexposure to the sun, you see no positive results, or you see a worsening or an irritation from what you're doing, that would be the time to get yourself to a dermatologist and have it checked out," says Dr. Novick.

The Sensitive Type

If your skin stings, itches and burns for seemingly no reason, you may have delicate skin. Here's what to do when your skin pitches a fit.

Do certain products burn, sting or cause a rash? Do you burn quickly without sunscreen? Does your face ever feel parched and fragile?

If you answered yes to one or more of the above questions, the chances are good that you have sensitive skin. Now, sensitivity may be great in a guy, but it's a lot less desirable when it comes to your complexion. And, alas, it's a lot more common—surveys taken in this country, Europe and Japan have found that almost 60 percent of women claim to suffer from the problem.

If the trend continues, sensitive skin is well on its way to becoming the PMS of the 1990s—a condition that afflicts many but remains stubbornly hard to pin down. Even doctors can't agree on a precise definition. Not to worry: All you really need to know is that we're using "sensitive skin" as an umbrella term to describe a variety of touchy skin situations. You may be irritated by ingredients that don't bother the rest of us. You may be allergic to something—and your body's immune system kicks in and fights back. You may be suffering a temporary skin setback—everything from pollution to heavy-duty treatment products can make even well-behaved skin go a little crazy. Whatever the cause, the results are similar: Your skin acts up—it gets itchy, scaly, red and blotchy; it burns or stings and sometimes it just *feels* that way without displaying visible symptoms. Bottom line: Something's wrong and you want to make it right. So before your complexion throws another fit, gain control by reading our pore-by-pore guide.

Genes may be partly to blame. If you have a family history of hay fever, asthma or eczema, your skin may be more irritable. Or, accord-

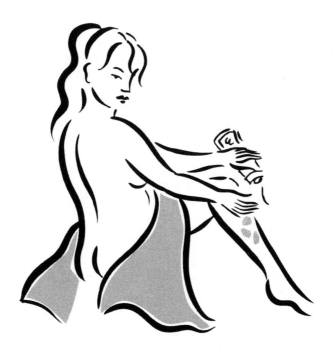

ing to Andrew J. Scheman, M.D., assistant clinical professor at North-western University Medical School in Chicago and co-author of *The Cosmetics Buying Guide*, you may have been born with thinner, more delicate skin, meaning your skin's natural defense barrier (made of lipids, the skin's built-in moisturizers) isn't up to performing its protective function. Rebecca James, instructor in cosmetic sciences at the University of California, Los Angeles, Extension, claims that "in cases of sensitive skin, there are holes in the lipids, and skin is actually more permeable." This is a double whammy, because on one hand, skin loses moisture; on the other, potentially irritating ingredients can creep in.

Coping with a Touchy Situation

If skin can't protect itself, it's up to you to step in and take charge. The best way to handle sensitive skin, experts agree, is by treating it as

---

CALMING STRESSED-OUT SKIN

The problem

fragile, delicate skin that can't stand up to harsh soaps; rough, grainy scrubs; alcohol-based toners and astringents.

---

fragrance-spooked skin that needs to avoid the obvious common-scents problems (and be wary of "unscented" as well).

---

very dry, irritated skin that cries out for super soothing.

---

sun-sensitive skin that needs protection from both the sun and potentially irritating sunscreens.

very dry skin. Don't scrub. Stay away from aggressive treatment products—for example, if you get very severe skin reactions, you should avoid the currently popular alpha hydroxy acids (if symptoms are mild, you might try one of the newer, less irritating versions, like Chanel Night Lift Plus). Sensitive skin needs sun protection, but only the gentlest kind. Some sunscreen ingredients, especially PABA, benzophenone and methoxycinnamate, cause allergic reactions and irritations. Look for products with titanium dioxide—a gentle, non-reactive physical sunblock that sits on the skin's surface. For specific treatment recommendations, see "Calming Stressed-Out Skin."

Avoiding Irritation

Almost anything, it seems, can cause sensitive skin to react. But the prime suspects in most cases of irritation include surfactants (the detergents used in soaps and cleansers), high levels of propylene glycol (a

---

The solution

kinder, gentler cleansers: Biomedic Gentle Cleansing Bar; Clinique Gentle Exfoliator; Guerlain Odely Instant Relaxing Cleanser; Repechage T-Zone Balance Cleansing Complex; Lancome Extremely Gentle Cream/Gel Cleanser.

products labeled "fragrance-free." Good examples: Dove Sensitive Skin Formula Beauty Bar; Almay Sensitive Care Eye Gel; Cuticura Medicated Antibacterial Bar Fragrance Free Formula for Sensitive Skin.

moisturizers with skin-friendly plant extracts or antioxidant formulas, including: Clarins Gentle Day Cream; Cabot's Multivitamin Facial Moisturizer for Sensitive Skin; Christian Dior Icone for Hyper-Sensitive Skins.

sun protectors with titanium dioxide, a gentle nonreactive physical sunblock. Try Origins and Estee Lauder Advanced Suncare products; Neutrogena No-Chemical Sunscreen.

moisturizing ingredient) and the alcohols used in toners and astringents. Allergic reactions tend to be triggered by fragrances and preservatives. Be wary of products labeled "unscented." This means that fragrance has been used to mask the natural scent of the ingredients. It *doesn't* mean fragrance-free, which is, in fact, exactly what you want.

When Skin Acts Up

What to do when, despite your best intentions, you use the wrong thing and get a bad case of the mean red itchies? First, give the area a cold-water rinse (for about 30 seconds). Your dermatologist may recommend a follow-up application of over-the-counter hydrocortisone cream. New rescue products include BeautiControl Skinlogics Corticure Comfort Lotion and Bioelements Immediate Comfort.

If you suffer strong—and frequent—reactions, a doctor may be able to prescribe antihistamines and steroidal anti-inflammatory creams.

The Next Best Thing

So what's ahead for sensitive types?

- New silicone-based ingredients that promise to moisturize skin and protect it from environmental hazards (another new class of protectors, perfluorochemicals, are currently being put to the test as a coating on the Taj Mahal).
- More vitamin-enriched products—especially those with A, C and E, which are known for their antioxidant properties. Why antioxidants? They're said to fight off environmental assaults—pollution, ultraviolet rays, secondhand smoke—while being kind to skin.
- "Green" treatments—primed with soothing plant extracts (look for kola, licorice, guarana, green tea) which manufacturers claim "stabilize" skin naturally.

More Than Just Mud

Facial masks can help hide fine lines as well as perform other youthifying (if temporary) feats. Here's a guide to these minor miracle workers.

The ancient Egyptians simply smeared mud all over their faces—an effective beauty ritual, but what did they know about pollution and sun damage? These days, the ingredients in masks are created for specific skin types and a myriad of skin problems—clogged pores, dryness, wrinkles, dullness—that your regular cleanser and moisturizer may not fully address. It's not easy to decipher the labels of many masks today, but it's essential to know what you're putting on your face and why.

"Masks should be used as an auxiliary to your regular routine," says Marianne Huss, vice-president of education at Clarins. "A mask is an intense treatment, delivering more than one can get out of a cleanser, toner or exfoliant." Call them little skin miracles: Masks do everything from diminishing the appearance of fine lines to clearing up acne to shedding the dull top layer of your skin. Because there are an overwhelming number to choose from (Do you need clay or mud? Deep-pore cleansing or peeling? Or how about one with alpha hydroxy acids?), the trick is to find the best one for your needs.

A Mask for Every Complexion

"The term *mask* is usually reserved for a product containing ingredients that form a barrier that traps perspiration at the skin surface, attracts water to the epidermis and exfoliates superficial skin cells," says Mary Lupo, M.D., a New Orleans-based dermatologist. In other words, a mask penetrates the skin to superhydrate your complexion while zapping dirt and dead skin cells away.

The oil-absorbing and hydrating versions tend to predominate, but there are masks formulated for every skin type and need. Even normal complexions can suffer from the occasional buildup of dead skin cells. "At least twice a year, you should re-evaluate your skin's condition. The mask that works wonders in the summer can dry out winter skin," says Huss. And even the oiliest complexion needs extra moisture in the winter months. No matter what type of mask you use, its effects will be temporary, according to Mark Goldgeier, M.D., a clinical assistant professor of dermatology at the University of Rochester in New York. "While richer ingredients and a longer exposure to the skin can allow masks to penetrate somewhat deeper, a topical solution like a mask really can't extend deep into the pores, so the effects will generally last only several hours," he says.

Spot-Toning Your Skin

Masks can also act as vehicles that allow ingredients like vitamins, alpha hydroxy acids and botanicals to enter the skin, Dr. Goldgeier adds. The extended exposure to the complexion allows these active elements to penetrate, and even after the mask is rinsed or peeled off, a residue will be left behind. But people with sensitive skin or allergies should take a close look at the ingredients list. "From a cosmetic point of view, it may be lovely to have essential oils or botanicals in the mask because they feel good and have pleasant odors," he says. "But from a medical point of view, they may increase the risk of an allergic reaction, both in themselves and because they also call for more preservatives." Formaldehydes and parabens, which are added to keep natural ingredients fresh, can often cause a stinging sensation or even a rash in touchy skins. Some masks contain mineral preservatives, but they must be refrigerated, and they last only for about two months.

Whether you're avoiding possible allergens or just trying to figure out what kind of results you'll get, a quick look at the label is always a good idea, says Barbara Salomone, director of education at Bioelements. "Even a mask for normal skin can have many different side benefits," she says. If you want a soothing preparation, look for ingredients like chamomile.

Although some masks are advertised as quick fixes for emerging skin disasters, experts recommend that a mask be used on a regular basis, generally once or twice a week. "It's kind of like exercising," says Salomone. "You really won't get the benefits if you use it only once every four months." Salomone tells her clients to reserve a half-hour each week, perhaps during their favorite television show. "The best way to apply the mask is to do a mini-facial," she says. "First cleanse your face, use a gentle exfoliant, then apply the mask and relax. After it's dry, rinse with warm water and a damp cloth, then apply moisturizer."

Take Your Pick—Clay, Mud or Gel

Most masks for oily skin are formulated with a base of clay. Spread all over the face (except the eye area), the clay hardens in 10 to 20 minutes, soaking up impurities and leaving the skin with a smooth feeling. When the mask is rinsed off, surface dirt, oil and dead skin cells adhere to the clay and are washed away with it. "These masks cause a slight inflammation which forces the pores closed so they appear smaller," says Dr. Goldgeier. "There also tends to be a redness, or 'healthy' glow." The drying effects of clay-based masks make them much too harsh for dry or sensitive skin types. (Remember, if your skin feels taut, it's a sign of overdrying, not squeaky cleanness.) To counteract the pure clay, many companies add soothing ingredients. Aveda's Deep Cleansing Herbal Clay Masque, for example, has echinacea, an herb with healing properties.

Like clay, mud masks soak up oil and leave the skin feeling super-clean—but mud's not as drying as clay, so it's easier on normal-to-oily complexions. Ahava's Mud Masque combines Dead Sea mud, waters and minerals to tone and tighten the skin without drying it out. Still, experts advise even people with normal skin to use clay or mud masks sparingly.

Combination skin types, with both dry patches and oily zones, are often the most difficult to address. The ideal solution is to use two masks, one on each region, but if that's a bother for you, try a gentle cleansing mask formulated for normal or combination skin. Many are in the form of a gel for easy application and contain active ingredients such as witch hazel, kaolin, titanium dioxide or bentonite, which remove excess dirt and oil but won't strip the skin of moisture. Spa Clear the Way Mask, a new entry from Elizabeth Arden, is a perfect example of the kind of mask that caters to combination skin types. Its oil-absorbing ingredients exfoliate and unclog pores while surfactants help wash away the impurities, according to Janet Bass, group leader for treatment and development at Elizabeth Arden. Also good is The Body Shop Peanut & Rosehip Face Mask, which combines cornstarch to cleanse, rose hips to condition and peanut oil to moisturize. (It also smells heavenly—nutty and sweet.)

Clear peel-off masks are ideal for combination skin; they work basically the same way as their rinse-away cousins. They are left on the face for 10 to 20 minutes and then rubbed or peeled off, removing dirt and dead skin cells. "Peel-off masks adhere to the impurities in skin and lift them off," says Lia Schorr, owner of the Lia Schorr Salon in New York City. Dr. Lupo cautions that the peeling action can be too hard on sensitive skin, although many contain calming ingredients: Chanel Blue Environmental Purifying Mask blends therapeutic aloe vera, chamomile and comfrey to calm environmentally abused skin and peel away dead cells.

Turning Dry Skin Dewy

Especially in the winter months, moisturizing masks can provide that extra boost of hydration that dry skin needs. Occlusive masks blend water and oils like glycerin, sorbitol or mineral oil, says Joan Osder, M.D., head of the Department of Dermatology at Century City Hospital in Los Angeles. They are "left on to trap moisture in the skin and not allow water to evaporate," she says.

Others, like Shiseido Vital-Perfection Hydro-Intensive Mask or Ultima II's 5-Minute Rehydrating Moisture Mask, saturate the skin to diminish fine lines. In general, these super-emollient masks do their work quickly; most of them are left on for three to ten minutes, tops. One warning, however: The intense creaminess of moisturizing masks can aggravate clogged pores and even ignite mini-breakouts, according to Dr. Lupo, so use them sparingly.

Alpha hydroxy acids (AHAs) are also showing up in facial masks. Touted for their ability to help slough off dead skin cells, AHAs work well on all but the most sensitive skin, says Dr. Osder. Some, like Clarins Perfecting Cream Mask, limit the percentage of fruit acids (to around 4 percent) to ensure surface-only exfoliation and reduce irritation, while others, like Dermalogica Gentle Cream Exfoliant, contain slightly higher amounts of lactic and salicylic acids for less sensitive skins. Since masks are left on for several minutes, they can be a good way to deliver AHAs to the skin, Dr. Osder says, but she recommends supplementing them with a daily dose of a moisturizer or any product that also contains alpha hydroxy acids.

Treat Your Skin to a Specialty Mask

Once you know the right type of mask for your skin, you can pamper yourself with one of the newer treatment masks.

Time-savers. Addressing the woman without the time for a full weekly facial is the goal of some of the latest masks on the market. Many companies are introducing ones that can do double duty—massaged in as a quick-fix scrub or moisturizer, or used more liberally, and then rinsed away like a regular mask. For dry skin, Prescriptives Flight Cream and Issima Aquamasque, from Guerlain, can be used as daily moisturizers or ten-minute facials. Three Minute Avocado Face Mask from Health & Beauty Farm by Bath & Body Works provides a fast moisture boost or can be left on extremely dry skin overnight.

Spot treatments. A new breed of mask hits the spots that need it most. Eye treatments, like Estee Lauder Stress Relief Eye Mask and Princess Marcella Borghese Formula Energia Eye Mask, contain restorative ingredients like comfrey that help reduce puffiness and make surface wrinkles less noticeable. DeCleor Contour Mask provides a three-minute fix for the eye area or the lips by smoothing and calming stressed and sensitive skin.

Emergency help. Acne masks, like Matrix Blemish Control Acne Treatment, help clear up existing breakouts and prevent future ones by soaking up oil and loosening blackheads. Neutrogena's Acne Mask contains 5 percent benzoyl peroxide for the kind of antibacterial control that promotes acne clear-ups. BeneFit Zinc Sulphur mask can be used as an overnight SOS treatment to reduce redness and make a pimple less noticeable, says BeneFit cofounder Jean Danielson. "People tend to ignore their skin, then get hysterical when there's a problem," she says. "Masks can be a comforting way to deal with any last-minute panic attacks."

PART SEVEN

Love and Intimacy

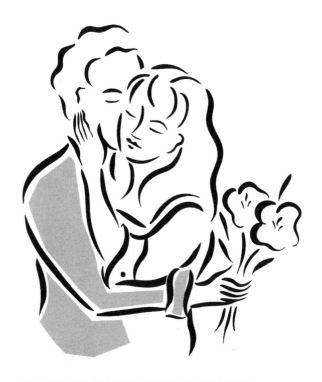

Never in the Mood?
Read This

You're just . . . not interested. But you're definitely not
alone. Here's how to overcome inhibited sexual desire.

*M*ovies, music videos, magazine articles and radio talk
shows send out a resounding message: sex, sex, sex.

Yet some women's bodies say no, no, no.

These women have inhibited sexual desire (ISD), a common disorder in which there is a chronic disinterest in sex. Forty to fifty percent of couples who show up at sexual dysfunction clinics are said to have it, making it the most common issue for couples who seek help for sexual problems.

Men are as likely as women to have it, says Richard A. Carroll, Ph.D., director of the Sex and Marital Therapy Program at the Northwestern Medical Faculty Foundation of the Northwestern Medical Center in Chicago. But women tend to get it at a younger age than men—in their midthirties as opposed to their fifties—and they tend to experience more emotional distress with it and go for longer periods of time without seeking help, he says.

Women with ISD experience more than just an occasional ebb in desire, says Jo Kessler, a licensed nurse practitioner and certified sex therapist in San Diego. These women can go for long periods of time—maybe six months, nine months, a year or longer—without feeling the urge. Some of them say they don't miss it at all, Kessler says. If it weren't for their partners, they wouldn't really care about having sex.

The situation can be a difficult one. With all the information about sex and sexuality that's available, women know that some amount of sex is considered "normal." "The woman knows if she's not having sex, or if she's not interested in sex, something is wrong. She feels defective, she feels guilty and she feels helpless," Kessler says. And if she perceives her partner as always ready to have sex, the woman may feel that she's the one with the problem and that she's totally to blame for the unsatisfactory sex life, she says.

What's Really Wrong

ISD is probably best thought of as a symptom of an underlying problem, says Dr. Carroll. The most common causes are more likely to be psychological than physical. At the top of the list is depression. "Depression can affect one's ability to enjoy anything. Sex is just one of those," he says.

Next in line is interpersonal conflict. Problems in a relationship often manifest themselves in sexual problems, experts say. "Sex is a metaphor for the relationship," says Susan E. Hetherington, Dr.P.H., a certified nurse-midwife and sex therapist and professor in the School of Nursing at the University of Maryland in Baltimore. "People end up fighting out in the bedroom what they should be fighting out in the living room and dining room," she says. When the couple doesn't deal with issues or problems by talking about them as they occur, the conflict comes out in other ways—often through the sexual relationship. Unexpressed anger is often part of the picture. With ISD, "in general the relationship isn't working or isn't providing the woman with what she wants or needs to be sexual," says Kessler.

The problem often develops gradually, she says. It may begin with a lack of enthusiasm for sex that causes the woman to decline sexual overtures sporadically, she says. Then, often without deliberately planning it as a sexual avoidance maneuver, the woman may get involved in activities that keep her chronically busy, unavailable or tired, so the likelihood of sex is reduced.

"Eventually a couple comes in and they haven't had sex for six months," she says. "The partner is frustrated and angry and upset. The woman is puzzled and upset and feeling pressured by her partner or by her own expectations. She's feeling overwhelmed. If she was depressed before, she's even more depressed. It can be a real downward spiral for the woman as well as for the relationship."

Physical changes, such as those occurring after pregnancy, might also trigger ISD. "It's not uncommon for a woman to be less interested in sex when there is a new baby at home. The woman is recovering physically and she's adapting to motherhood. All of the demands that having a new baby put on a woman contribute to fatigue," says Kessler. Often women will have a lower sex drive for six to nine months after having a baby, she says.

Despite common belief, women going through menopause won't automatically experience ISD. "If she's had a healthy sex drive and a healthy attitude about sex and has liked it and it's been a positive force in her life, unless there's some untoward problem with the menopause, it doesn't really affect her drive at all," says Kessler. "There used to be the notion that when women got older or went through menopause they lost interest in sex, and that's just not holding true." The sex drive of some women actually goes up after menopause, she says. "There can be such a sense of freedom that women are more interested sexually. Some report it as the best sexual time of their life."

Keeping Desire Strong

ISD can be prevented. Here's what you can do.

Pay attention to problems. "Have some mechanism to resolve conflict in the relationship. When couples are fighting, they don't feel particularly congenial," says Kessler, and they usually won't want to have sex. Instead of letting one issue color the whole relationship and all your interactions, set aside a specific time to address it. "For example, talk about the issue for 30 minutes, then set it aside. Agree that you'll do that every second or third day for two weeks and that at two weeks you'll have formed some resolution. That's one way to keep it from constantly being up in your face and being the total focus of your relationship with each other," she says.

Keep the lines of communication open. When you are upset, try to deal with the problems instead of pushing them under the rug, says Dr. Hetherington. Try using "I" statements and avoid using "you" statements, she says. Start with "I feel this way" or "I am frustrated," instead of "You make me mad." Another way to express and defuse feelings of anger or resentment is to write them out first, says Dr. Carroll. Then figure out how you can relay the message in an effective way, he says.

Initiate intimacy. Couples need to set aside time to be together in an intimate way, says Dr. Carroll. "Set one night aside to be together—alone—without the kids or distractions. Make a commitment to time for the relationship," he says.

Vary your sexual routine. Try new things with your partner to keep from getting in the same old habit. "People with ISD have fairly rigid sexual scripts. This is how sex is done—A, B, C and D," says Dr. Carroll. "A varied sexual repertoire can help prevent ISD."

Think about sex. "One way to keep sex drive alive is thinking about sex. Have three erotic thoughts a day, from mildly romantic to whatever any individual woman thinks of as sexually explicit," says Kessler. "If you don't ever think about sex, then it's not very likely that you're going to keep your appetite stimulated. It's important for a woman to help get herself in the mood," she says. Having some romantic or sexual thoughts during the day can serve as a kind of warm-up for sex later that night, she says.

Renew That Loving Feeling

If you have ISD or think you may be developing it, experts have some suggestions.

Take time to touch. One way to stay physically close when desire is low is to defocus from intercourse and orgasm and refocus on more generalized touching of the body, says Kessler. No breasts or genitals at first; wait until you are *both* ready before you include those parts. Set aside periods twice a week when you and your partner spend up to half an hour touching each other in affectionate, nonsexual ways. Do this in a room that's warm and relaxed, and perhaps light candles or play a tape to augment the mood. Be sure to talk to each other, too, expressing feelings.

"Use a touch with no sexual expectations or demands in the beginning," she says. "The idea is for each to get comfortable with themselves and their partner's bodies, not immediately turn each other on." The "turn-on" will follow as you learn how to "tune in" first, she says.

Put yourself in the mood. Try reading romantic novels or short stories that you like that have a romantic story line, says Kessler. Or rent a movie geared toward sensuality. "Find a love story you like that will create the mood" for sex for you, she says.

Schedule a "sex date." If a woman's desire is low and she's not too interested in sex, she may avoid her partner for fear that if she touches or kisses him, it will be interpreted as an overture for sex, says Kessler. If the couple sets a time when they both agree to have sex, that can take the pressure off. The woman will feel free to kiss or touch her partner affectionately at other times and know it won't have to lead to sex. And "making a date for sex can be a lot of fun," she says.

Get help early. If you feel that you're starting to have problems, take care of it sooner rather than later, says Dr. Carroll. "If it goes on a long time, it's likely to get worse," he says. Consult with a neutral third party, says Kessler. You might try calling a therapist who specializes in sexual dysfunction and asking if what you're experiencing sounds like something you should be worried about, she says. When you decide on therapy, ideally both partners should be involved, says Kessler.

Recapturing the Passion

If the sizzle has fizzled, take heart. It's possible to rediscover better-than-ever loving—even with the same partner.

Ever since the birth of their son Brian, Janet and Ted Flagman saw their sex life slipping away. Between raising Brian and his younger sister, Anna, and holding down a part-time job, Janet could barely muster enough energy to watch television—much less schedule a passionate interlude with Ted, who was equally exhausted from climbing the corporate ladder all day. "We've always joked that our romance would return when the kids went to college," says Janet. "But three years have passed since Anna left the nest, and that spark is as elusive as ever. Now we're afraid we're simply too old for a passionate love life."

Janet and Ted's experience with waning sexual desire isn't uncommon. And neither is their concern that as gray hairs emerge, desire fades. Fortunately, according to the experts, their worries are unfounded. In a study conducted at Duke University in Durham, North Carolina, researchers found that eight out of ten men in their late sixties continue to be sexually active. And according to similar studies, women also retain their interest in sex throughout their lifetimes. So if you're experiencing a sexual slowdown, don't give up hope. You can regain the desire that seems to be lost. And the first step is figuring out why passion fled in the first place.

Why the Sizzle Fizzles

Passion is sensitive to everything from changes in hormones to changes in climate. According to sex therapist Michael Seiler, Ph.D., associate director of the Phoenix Institute in Chicago and co-author of *ISD: Inhibited Sexual Desire*, passion is "a psychosomatic experience," a shivery response by your body to some delightful tickle in your head. This response is easily triggered by anything from a weekend getaway with your lover to a spouse who brings you breakfast in bed and cleans up afterward. And unfortunately, it's just as easily quelled. Here are a few of the top causes of a flagging libido.

Anger. Many experts believe that unresolved anger in a relationship is the primary cause of decreased sex drive. The anger may come from anywhere—"He never tells me he loves me" or "He never puts his dirty socks in the hamper." But in a two-career family, it often comes down to division of labor. For example, if a woman continues to work and do the majority of the household chores after she and her husband have children, she may feel overwhelmed and alone. Instead of simply asking her husband to pitch in, she shoulders the burden alone and begins resenting her spouse. And when a woman is angry or hurt, she's unlikely to feel frisky.

"For a woman, sex isn't about how her partner touches her body. It's about how he touches her psyche—how he relates to her within the context of their relationship," says Dr. Seiler. "Feeling connected and cared for is what turns on women most."

Stress. It comes with birth and death, beginnings and endings, rises and falls in fortune—and it may be your libido's second-biggest enemy. The fact is, many couples are so busy with work, the house and the daily pressures of living that they don't set aside time for each other. "We leave passion behind when we focus too much attention on things that aren't related to the pleasure we feel with our partners," says Sandra R. Scantling, Psy.D., assistant clinical professor of psychiatry at the University of Connecticut School of Medicine in Farmington and co-author of *Ordinary Women, Extraordinary Sex*.

Fear. Sexual desire flourishes only when a woman feels safe and secure. If sex makes you anxious in any way, you'll want it about as much as you want an IRS audit. Some women are afraid of letting themselves be swept away by their own passion. "They think, 'What's he going to say if I yell, scream or moan?' " says Judith Seifer, Ph.D., R.N., president of the American Association of Sex Educators, Counselors and Therapists. "Fear is a profound inhibitor of sexual desire; it's hard to let go if you're inhibited."

Other women fret that they're not doing it right, as if each sexual encounter was a pop quiz that counted toward a final grade. And still others are afraid to discuss their sexual needs with their partners. When we ask and don't get a positive response, we stop asking, and we withdraw. Then we wonder why sex doesn't happen anymore.

Hints for Better Sex

The good news is that no matter what has driven the desire away, if you once felt those erotic urges, you can feel them again. But don't expect miracles overnight. "There are no 'three easy steps to a better sex life,' " says Leslie Schover, Ph.D., clinical psychologist at the Center for Sexual Function at the Cleveland Clinic. "Sexual desire is complex. What helps one person may not do anything for the next." With this caveat in mind, take note of the following expert advice on how to reignite your sexual fire.

Get a checkup. There's a myriad of causes for sexual dysfunction and loss of desire—and some of them are medical in nature. Menopause, medications, diseases and illnesses all can cause a loss of sexual desire or lead to painful intercourse.

Get moving. Exercise has long been recommended to improve health, increase longevity and maintain a healthy weight. But regular aerobic exercise strengthens the heart and lungs, energizes the body and tones the muscles, too. All of these factors contribute to improved self-esteem as well as better physical endurance in any activity—including sex.

Get your man moving, too. Engaging in regular aerobic exercise may help boost a man's performance in bed. In one study, a group of 78 previously inactive men began a program of jogging or bicycling three times a week for an hour a day. After nine months, these men reported a 30 percent increase in frequency of intercourse and 26 percent more orgasms than before they began the workout program.

What's more, if you and your partner begin exercising together (such as following the walking program in "Do the Stroll," page 198), you'll be increasing the amount of time you spend together—an important factor in any intimate relationship.

Take your time. Sexual response slows down a bit with age. A woman's ovaries produce less estrogen after menopause, which causes the lining of the vagina to become thinner and to secrete less lubricating mucus during sexual arousal. This means that you may need more foreplay in preparation for making love, and that you may want to use a lubricating jelly. Men secrete less testosterone as they age, so erections take longer to develop and may be less firm. So slow down—getting there is half the fun!

Schedule your interludes. You and your partner need to make time for one another, even if it means scheduling time for sex. "People will say, 'Oh, no—that's so predictable, so unspontaneous,' " says Lonnie Barbach, Ph.D., assistant clinical professor of psychotherapy at the University of California, San Francisco, School of Medicine. "Our calendars are full, and if we don't pencil in sex, the time will get filled with something else."

Spend time together. It's as important to schedule talking time as it is to schedule sex. Go out to dinner, see a play or get away for a weekend. Then, when you're together, talk to each other about your job, your life, your childhood and your dreams. Ask your partner questions about his ideas, beliefs and desires, and encourage him to do the same. Even if you've been together for years, you'll be surprised at how many new things you'll learn about your partner simply by talking.

Talk out your troubles. "Sexual intercourse rarely occurs without verbal discourse," says Dr. Seiler. But like many people, you may find it easier to avoid sex than to discuss it. And you may have just as much trouble airing other, seemingly mundane grievances, as well.

To keep your discussions of sensitive topics from turning into battles, don't put your partner on the defensive. Use "I" statements rather than "you" statements. "I" statements describe how you feel; "you" statements sound like accusations.

Keep talking. One discussion, no matter how successful, isn't going to cure what's ailing your love life. So plan for regular powwows. If you try talking things over without success, your best bet may be to seek the help of a marriage counselor or a certified sex therapist.

Communicate your desires. Tell your partner exactly what you want—in bed and out. Your biggest turn-on might be seeing your partner voluntarily cleaning the bathroom. Or it might be a certain way he touches your breasts. Or both. Tell him. And ask him to share his desires with you, too.

Explore your sensual side. To start, Dr. Scantling suggests identifying something that makes you feel good. Remember a romantic getaway. Reread old love letters, listen to soothing music or fantasize about sex. Give yourself time each day to experience and savor these pleasant sensations.

Explore your sexual side. Many therapists recommend watching erotic movies or reading books on sex. Your local bookstore is likely to have half a dozen books on sexual technique, many of which are illustrated. Or if you'd rather be more discreet about such purchases, you can order them by mail (in a plain brown wrapper, of course).

Allow yourself to fantasize. In her research, Dr. Scantling found that women who enjoy fantasy reported much higher sexual enjoyment and arousal. Fantasies of people other than your partner—both real and imagined—are natural and normal, too, she adds.

Romance each other. Dr. Barbach advises her clients to court each other as if they were dating. Write each other poems and love notes. Buy little presents for no special reason. Send flowers. Pitch in with chores. Phone just to say "I love you." Reaching out in these little ways will help bring you closer.

MASSAGE: RUB HIM THE RIGHT WAY

*I*f you've been with your lover for years, you may find that physical contact has been reduced to a daily peck on the cheek and an occasional session of lovemaking that ends in orgasm only minutes after it began. Fortunately, it's never too late to learn new ways of touching, and massage can help you do just that. Here's how to give a sensual massage.

Set the mood. Select a place where you won't be interrupted. Take the phone off the hook. Lock the door. Forget about time. If you like, play some relaxing music and dim the lights.

Smooth on some oil. You can buy expensive massage oils at novelty shops or through catalogs, but ordinary safflower or coconut oil work fine, too. It's best to warm the oil, then test its temperature on your skin before applying it to your partner's.

Go from head to toe. Begin by massaging the forehead, jaw muscles and temples, then move down, leaving no skin untouched. When you reach the feet, spend a good deal of time deeply massaging them, especially if your partner spends a lot of time standing.

Ask for feedback. People tend to touch others in the way they like to be touched. This means men rub too firmly and women, too gently. To avoid this, keep asking your partner, "How does this feel?" Then alter your touch to please him.

Just say no. To sex, that is—at least until you've finished the massage. This means you shouldn't touch the genitals until you've covered the rest of the body. The reason for this seeming contradiction? Postponing lovemaking helps build sexual tension. So when you finally do make love, it's likely your encounter will be more intense than it has been in years.

Switch roles. Now it's your turn to be pampered.

Remember the good times. No matter how great you have it, your relationship inevitably will encounter stormy seas. When that happens, remind yourself (and your partner) of all of the smooth sailing you've experienced—and all the good times that lie ahead. Together, you can weather the storm.

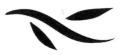

Every Man's Nightmare

*One man shares what it's like to experience a
"false start" in the sack—and lets us in on what
we can do to help.*

*I*t's a measure of the penis's prominence—its unparalleled importance in lovemaking and in life—that when The Big Guy fails to
measure up to expectations in bed, well, life in general seems a little
limp, too.

We men want to be assembly-not-required, ready-at-a-moment's-
notice kind of guys—all the time. But we know better. Because gravity strikes all men at least once. Believe me: We're all too aware of the
fact that Mr. Happy sometimes falls down on the job—or worse,
never even shows up.

Our doctors tell us that one out of every 10 men over the age of
21—about 30 million in all—has trouble getting it up on a chronic
basis. And that millions more experience erectile dysfunction, as it's
called, once or twice in their lifetimes. Still, we are not soothed.

Maybe you know all this already. Maybe your partner's had trouble getting an erection once or twice. Or perhaps it's happened a few
times in a row and he's now reluctant to initiate sex altogether. And
you're worried. About your relationship, your sex appeal.

Relax. I can tell you this: Most likely, there's nothing wrong with
your guy that a little prodding and some special attention won't cure.
Pay close attention. I'll tell you what to do . . . .

How a Man Operates

You wouldn't know unless someone told you, but getting an erection is pretty tricky business. Standard operating procedure is as follows: When a man becomes aroused, nerve impulses send messages to
the muscles surrounding two arteries, both of which feed into highly
elastic cylinders (the corpora cavernosa) made of erectile tissue that
runs the length of the penis. The muscles respond by relaxing their
grip on the arteries, which allow the cylinders to fill with blood. The

result is a thick, rigid penis, primed for penetration and ejaculation.

Sometimes, however, not everything goes according to plan. A message is misrouted, a signal lost. And it's strikeout city.

As you might expect, erectile dysfunction is more likely to occur with age. Middle-age and older men who suffer from heart problems and diabetes frequently report having trouble getting a rise out of The Big Guy (largely because of the restricted circulation usually associated with these conditions). In addition, erectile difficulty is common among men taking blood pressure or ulcer medications, which can inhibit blood flow to the penis and slow an erection. Illegal drugs, alcohol and cigarette smoking can lower the boom, too.

In many cases, however—especially when you're talking about the average, red-blooded, healthy male—an elusive erection has its roots in the mind, not the body. "It's extremely rare for men below the age of 50, who are otherwise in good health, to experience erectile difficulties because of a physical problem or illness," says Joshua Golden, M.D., clinical professor of psychiatry and former director of the Human Sexuality Program at the University of California, Los Angeles.

This being the case, you're in a great position (no pun intended) to help out should Mr. Happy become a bit depressed. Here's how.

Do some detective work. Before you dismiss the possibility that your partner's erectile problems are physical in nature, ask yourself the following questions: Does he often wake up with an erection? Does he get erections during the night? When you're hugging, kissing and fondling each other, does he get and maintain an erection? Does he get an erection when he masturbates? (You may have to do some digging to get an answer to this one.) Has his problem developed suddenly?

If you can answer "yes" to all or most of the above, your partner's problem probably isn't physical, says Perry Nadig, M.D., clinical professor of urologic surgery at the University of Texas Health Sciences Center in Austin. If your man's capable of getting an erection, his penis is probably fit for duty. Similarly, a man who can bring himself to orgasm solo should be physically capable of doing so with his partner.

The sudden inability to maintain an erection under very specific circumstances—such as during penetration—often indicates a psychological problem. Physical impediments to erectile function generally develop gradually, and they affect men consistently, whereas psychologically triggered erectile problems frequently develop overnight and are sporadic.

If you think your partner's problem may be physical, talk to him about seeing a urologist, who can recommend a whole host of treatments, from drug therapy to penile vascular surgery. For more treatment information, call the Impotence Institute of America at 1-800-669-1603. Counselors there can refer you to experts and help you understand the physiological and psychological ramifications of erectile dysfunction.

Put yourself in his shoes. Sex is generally very penis-oriented for men. "When a man thinks about sex," says Dr. Golden, "he's focusing on getting an erection, how hard it's going to be and how long it's going to last."

Women, on the other hand, generally don't define sex so narrowly, says Dr. Nadig. Yes, women desire actual intercourse just as much as men do. But most women are also more apt to think about sex in a larger sense.

For instance, you probably consider kissing, foreplay and post-penetration snuggling all part of a single pleasure package. We don't. So if we fall down on the job, you might still consider that you've had sex. We don't.

Understand, too, that a false start isn't forgotten when you both decide to call it quits, roll over and get some shut-eye. After a man has a performance problem—even just once—he may begin to obsess over whether it will happen repeatedly. And when we apply that kind of pressure, it's tough to produce—much less maintain—an erection.

What can you do? For starters, suggest ways in which your partner can please you without using his penis—whether it's bringing you to orgasm with his hands or giving you an all-body massage. Be creative. "The less you need an erect penis for an enjoyable sexual experience," says Dr. Golden, "the more likely you are to get one."

Get him talking. There's nothing like stress coupled with low self-esteem to deflate a man's, um, enthusiasm. So encourage your partner to share his worries, fears and frustrations, and—even more important—remind him why you find him so sexy.

Maybe he's feeling self-conscious about the spare tire that re-

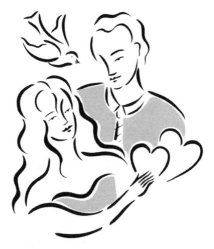

cently staked a claim around his middle. Perhaps his job's been awful, his boss a jerk. So ask him how he's doing—and really listen to what he tells you. Then later, when the lights are low, regale him with a blow-by-blow account of the best, most exciting sex you've ever had with him. Tell him exactly what he does to make you squirm and shudder with delight. In other words, stroke his ego—and his erection.

Resist pointing fingers. Chances are, if your partner's feeling sexually inadequate, he's also feeling defensive. So take special care not to assign blame when you discuss your sexual problems, even though you, too, may be feeling frustrated.

"Try not to view your sexual problems in terms of what one person is or isn't doing for the other person," advises psychologist Sallie Schumacher, Ph.D., former president of the American Association of Sex Educators, Counselors and Therapists. "Most people become anxious when they feel they're being accused. And that only prompts them to lash back."

Relieve the pressure. "Sex is yet another life category in which men feel they're expected to excel," says Janet Wolfe, Ph.D., executive director of the Institute for Rational-Emotive Therapy in New York City and author of *What to Do When He Has a Headache: Renewing Desire and Intimacy in Your Relationship*. Since no one—not even your guy—can perform up to snuff all the time, undue pressure can spell disaster in the bedroom.

How can you relieve your star player's jitters? Easy: Let him know that you don't expect him to hit a home run every time he steps up to the plate—that all you're really looking for is unconditional closeness. No pressure. No performing.

"Start by encouraging only cuddling and caressing—no genital stimulation," says Dr. Wolfe. "In time, your partner will begin to relax, which may be just enough to get him going again—on his own terms."

Whip him into shape. A tired, wired body is a body primed for erectile failure. The proper prescription? Exercise. Working out eases tension and strengthens the body, which increases a man's odds of being able to become sexually aroused. So hop to it with your partner. Walk the dog together. Join a gym together. Take the stairs together. Use this opportunity to get in shape—and to get closer.

In addition, encourage your guy to substitute water, a soft drink or a nonalcoholic beer for his nightly brew. Alcohol dulls the body's responses and can chase away a man's erections. The same goes for smoking, which constricts blood vessels and squeezes off circulation.

Finally, if your guy's not getting enough rest, his libido may be tired, too. Try to get eight hours of shut-eye a night. Better yet, hit the sheets early—together.

Recreate romance. You can't just leap into bed together and expect the magic to be there—automatically—15 years, a few kids and a hefty mortgage after you've said "I do." You have to plan. So invite your guy to take a Saturday afternoon nap with you, then wake up refreshed—and make love. Rent a sexy movie and watch it in your bedroom—naked. Surprise him at breakfast—as breakfast. In short, set the scene and remind him that when it comes to making love, only fools rush in.

A Better Way to Argue

He's the king of the cheap shot, and his fighting style is wearing you out. Here's a smarter way to iron out your differences.

Charlotte (suspiciously): *When* did you tell me?

Bill: While you were on the phone yakking with your sister. The trouble is, you'd forget your head if it wasn't screwed on. And, by the way, the broccoli was overcooked.

Charlotte: I can't believe this. How dare you criticize me like that after what you've just put me through!

And so it goes. Many women, alas, can identify all too well with the above scenario. "About 98 percent of the time Bill is the sweetest man on Earth," Charlotte confides. "But when we fight he throws out zingers that hurt me for weeks. Once when I was trying to discuss my frustrations with our sex life, he shouted, 'Well, you've gained weight, and it turns me off!' I was devastated. Why can't he fight nice?"

Zingers are merely *one* way men fight dirty. Other ploys include:

Distracting you from the real issue. "Okay, so I didn't phone when I promised. But what about that time your mother insulted me at dinner and you didn't stick up for me?"

Questioning your motives. "I don't think where we go on vacation is the issue here. You just don't want me to have fun."

Denying your feelings. "You're not really upset with me because I ignore you; you're upset because my career is going well and you're frustrated and stagnating in yours."

Blaming you. After he says something mean and you react, he blames you by saying, "You're too sensitive."

What can you do with a man like this? First, you can try to figure out where he's coming from.

Do Men Experience Anger Differently?

If your mate gets more worked up than you do during a quarrel, it might be because many men experience more intense physical reactions to conflict than women. In his studies of spouses discussing unresolved issues, psychology professor Clifford Notarius, Ph.D., of Catholic University of America in Washington, D.C., found that even when the husbands appeared calm and collected, they triggered notable responses on a biofeedback machine. These physical responses may make it more difficult for men to control their reactions when angry (or more likely to die of heart attacks!).

And how we react when we're angry is key. According to Carol Tavris, Ph.D., author of *Anger: The Misunderstood Emotion*, while men and women feel and express anger with about the same frequency, they react in different ways. Men respond more angrily to "ego insults" (criticism) than women do. When a man's ego is threatened, he's likely to erupt in anger, whereas a woman is more apt to act hurt (to sulk or cry). Men are also likelier than women to express anger in public. Dr. Tavris says, "Both sexes may feel annoyed or angry with a nervy fellow who cuts ahead of them in a movie line . . . but men are more willing to say or do something about it."

Why Does He Say Such Dreadful Things?

The fact that men express anger differently still doesn't justify why a man who swears he loves you may call you a "moron" in the heat of an argument. Sure, later he may plead, "Why can't you just forgive and forget? You know I didn't mean it." But you may not be so sure. What if his nasty remark reflects what he really feels? Besides, what if you said the same kind of stuff to him? He would go crazy!

"What a man shouts in anger during a quarrel often shouldn't be taken too personally," insists Joseph Nowinski, Ph.D., a psychologist in Mansfield, Connecticut. "From the time they're little boys, males in our culture are taught it's okay to fight dirty—as long as you win."

Of course, women fight down and dirty sometimes, but most women agree that men seem far more likely to do so. Truth is, a man who spits out nasty remarks on a regular basis has often modeled his behavior after his father. When his mother confronted his father for buying a top-of-the-line car without consulting her, his father may have exploded, "It's hopeless trying to talk to you about this. You just get ir-

THE KNOCK-DOWN-DRAG-OUT FIGHT

*E*very couple occasionally has a fight so hideous shoes are flung and the obscenities fly. Well, can the guilt. All-out, in-your-face fights are not only normal, they may even be necessary from time to time. But the question is: How far should you go?

Most women agree that it's not how terrible your fights are that matters most, it's what you do when they're over. If you both resort to sulking and skulking around afterward, that's deadly. You both have to admit that something scary happened, you're both responsible and you have to forgive each other.

Still, there are limits. As one woman says, "My husband and I agree never to say anything irrevocably hurtful. I can't have children, and he would never use that against me. I think that's important—to agree where the line is."

Most of us can't and shouldn't tolerate personal attacks like, "You're so fat I can't stand to look at you." Make them forbidden. One woman also suggests outlawing anything that questions the marriage itself. "It's not okay to say, 'I wish I weren't married to you,' " she says. "If you say those things to each other you will never feel safe in the relationship again."

Finally, most women agree, set a time limit for your fury: Any fight that lasts longer than a day has lasted too long.

rational when you have PMS." So when you complain about something, your mate may automatically use the same line against you.

When He Feels He Has the Right to Fight Nasty

Charlotte says, "What bothers me most is Bill's attitude that he somehow has the right to say this stuff. No matter how angry I get I'd never tell him he's not sexy. So why does he assume he can say that to me?"

The answer? Often we only feel safe insulting people we regard as lower in status than ourselves. "Most people have difficulty expressing anger to others of higher status," says Dr. Tavris. So if he can talk about your cellulite but you would never dare mention his paunch, you need to ask this: Are you truly "equal" in this relationship?

FOUR TYPES OF DIRTY FIGHTERS

The Public Offender. When you're alone, he's all sugar-and-spice. Then at a party he'll blurt out your most embarrassing secret. How to respond? Don't play his game. After the party, when he pretends he was just joking and says you're "overreacting," tell him you know what he's up to and you want him to stop.

The Intimidator. He tries to keep you "one down" in the relationship by raising his voice, slamming doors or threatening to leave. Stand quietly firm. Once he realizes you won't be bullied, he'll have to talk.

The Put-Down Artist. Tell him you forgot to pick up his shirts at the laundry, and he'll say you have "a mind like a sieve." Dealing with this type requires knowing your own worth and refusing to let him undermine it.

The Brooder. When you fail to fulfill his wishes (making love when he wants to, going to the movie he prefers), he withdraws into stony silence. Resist trying to coax him out of his "mad." Let him sulk until he's ready to express his needs directly—as an adult.

In fact, if *either* of you resorts to personal attacks during a quarrel, pay attention. When University of Southern California researchers studied 73 couples, they found that those with strong marriages were able to fight constructively even during heated battles. "They may have shouted at each other, but at the peak of their anger they also expressed warmth, even humor," says psychology professor Gayla Margolin, Ph.D., who headed the study. "They didn't just insult and blame each other, they offered solutions."

Keep His Anger from Hurting Your Love

If you're involved with a dirty fighter, what can you do? First, if a man continually makes jokes at your expense, derides your opinions or has you straining to be "perfect" to keep from triggering his rage, he's worse than unfair, he's abusive, and you may want to question the future of the relationship. If your normally nice Joe occasionally fights nasty, however, consider these tips.

Don't hold anger in. When you can, try to agree that when either of you feels hurt, you'll quickly speak up. Too often we're taught to believe we can save a relationship by staying silent and keeping the peace. But according to John Gottman, Ph.D., a marriage researcher at the University of Washington in Seattle, one of the most damaging behaviors in a marriage is sulking withdrawal—especially on the part of the man.

Tell him how you feel. As Dr. Gottman points out, when contempt is displayed in even the briefest facial expression—like his rolling his eyes upward or sneering while you're talking to him—it can be every bit as powerful a put-down as saying, "You're stupid." Don't put up with his nasty tone of voice, either.

Refuse to be distracted. If you're trying to discuss your need for more sexual foreplay and he replies, "How can you expect me to feel sexy when you wear that dowdy old nightgown to bed," calmly acknowledge his feelings ("Maybe I do need some new lingerie . . . "), then get back to the real issue ("but we're talking here about the lack of equality in our love life").

Be the bigger mate. As unfair as it is, University of Washington researchers have found that in happy marriages the women generally break the argument cycle in the most intense conflicts. She may interject a note of humor or even respond positively ("Well, I don't care what you say: I still love you").

Tell him to think, then talk. Insist that he control his anger. Remind him of the times you've thought of saying hurtful things but held your tongue, and ask that he take a 30-minute "time-out."

Forgive him. When you forgive your mate rather than hold a grudge, you're saying, "I'm self-sufficient enough to choose you even though you sometimes make mistakes that hurt me." And that's one of the key signs of mature love.

PART EIGHT

Stress Control

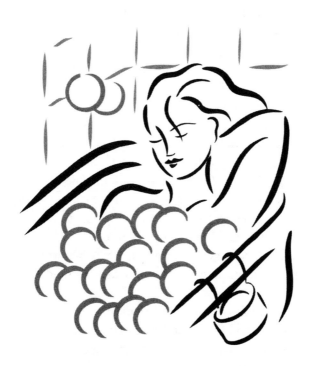

Escape the Do-It-All Syndrome

Too much stress can tax your immune system
as well as your sanity. Here's advice to help you
regain some much-needed serenity.

At 37, Fran Davis was the quintessential Philadelphia lawyer. She worked 80 hours a week, traveled from one case to another all over the country, worked on some of the biggest and hottest cases in corporate America and loved every minute of it.

"I was a born litigator," she says. "I have a real go-for-the-jugular thing about lawyering. It's exciting and it's exhilarating. Yes, it's stressful. But I don't look at stress as a negative word. I need a certain amount to do what I want to do, to be competitive."

Unfortunately, she adds dryly, "it tends to get out of hand." Stress can build until, rather than giving you an edge, it becomes destructive. You lose your concentration, forget things and start to get disorganized.

All this happened to Fran Davis. But she's not the only woman to let stress get out of hand.

Seventy-five percent of women and 70 percent of men between the ages of 25 and 44 say they experience "a lot" or a "moderate amount" of stress in their lives, according to a survey conducted by the National Center for Health Statistics in Hyattsville, Maryland.

And a study by the Northwestern National Life Insurance Company in Minneapolis reported that more than half of the workers in high-stress jobs suffer from physical or mental problems such as exhaustion, insomnia and headaches. Further, women seem particularly affected. Not only are they more likely to report stress-related illness, they are more likely to feel burned out and think about quitting.

In a survey by the Families and Work Institute in New York, 40 percent of women said they found it hard to get up and face another day at work every morning, and 42 percent said they feel "used up" by the end of the day.

Why are so many women burned out, used up and stressed out? Hormones, evolving social roles and a national marketplace that's reinventing itself are some good guesses. And unlike Fran Davis, who reduced her litigation work, cut her hours in half, moved to the country and worked from home, most women—particularly those with families to support—can't take such radical steps to reduce stress.

The Survival Advantage

The way our bodies respond to stress is preprogrammed. It's an ancient survival mechanism, genetically transmitted from generation to generation, that has kept our species on the alert for centuries.

When the senses perceive any threat to our existence, the brain triggers a flood of chemicals throughout the body—primarily epinephrine, norepinephrine and adrenocorticotropin—that will prepare it to fight or flee. The heart beats faster, more oxygen gets to the muscles, energy from fat and sugar is released, blood clotting speeds up and immune responses slow down.

In turn, adrenocorticotropin also triggers the release of the hormone cortisol, which essentially maintains this turbocharged state as long as the threat exists.

But although a woman's stress response works in much the same way as a man's, there are some major factors that make her response to stress far stronger, says researcher Eva Redei, Ph.D., assistant professor of pharmacology and psychiatry at the University of Pennsylvania in Philadelphia.

"Women naturally have higher levels of cortisol than men," she explains. Dr. Redei's animal studies indicate that the female hormone estrogen also increases a woman's chemical response to stress. Significant changes in levels of progesterone, another female sex hormone, alter the stress response the same way that cortisol does. Our levels of progesterone increase eight to ten times just before we menstruate.

"These changes in stress responses are like riding a roller coaster," says Dr. Redei. They give women a survival advantage in terms of their ability to sense danger and react within a heartbeat. The problem is that a woman's stress response system can't tell the difference between a deadline-intense project at work, an injured child at home and a marauding dinosaur. It just goes to full alert at the drop of a hat—raising our levels of stress and dampening our immune system just enough to make us vulnerable to everything from colds, cancer and heart disease to inflammatory bowel disease, diabetes and asthma.

Let Him Help

Although studies indicate that the complexity of women's roles—worker, wife, mother, daughter, friend—actually acts as a buffer against stress from any single role, trying to deal with the sheer number of tasks that are involved in these roles can produce enough stress to sink a ship.

But do we ask for help?

Not on your life. "We think we need to do it all on our own," says therapist Mandy Manderino, Ph.D., associate professor at the University of Missouri in Columbia.

Not only do we need to be the perfect wife and mom, we need to be the perfect employee as well.

"It's important for women to stop overfunctioning and ask for help," she adds. "Some women are beginning to discover they need not do it all. However, other women continue to try to be everything to everyone. It is these women who are at high risk for stress-related problems."

Here's what you can do to get some much-needed help.

Set your priorities. Of all the myriad tasks demanding your attention, ask yourself which is the most important. Your daily to-do list should be based on your personal goals, says Dr. Manderino. "Is an absolutely spotless toilet bowl a top priority for you?" she asks. "Or is it more important to go out in the yard and play baseball with your kids or perhaps finish your college degree?"

Get off the back burner. "Oftentimes women put themselves last or leave themselves out entirely when setting priorities. They have difficulty making time for themselves," says Dr. Manderino. They can just never get to the gym or find a half-hour to soak in the tub. "They say, 'Well, I'd like to, but all these other things come first.'

"But if you're giving away energy, there has to be a way to get back energy," she points out. "There has to be some 'me' time. And if that constantly gets moved to please someone else, you're going to continue to be stressed."

Pick a time every day and set it aside to do things just for yourself, says Dr. Manderino. Play, relax, exercise—do anything you like. But it can't be unpleasant work, and it can't be for anybody else but you.

Re-energize. Fight stress by renewing your personal energy with some type of relaxation exercise, says Dr. Manderino. Do yoga, tai chi or meditation—whatever works for you.

"I'm a really active person, and I can't meditate," says Dr. Manderino. "I can't sit still. So I do a walking meditation. I walk and focus on the 'now.' I anchor myself in the present by trying to notice the wildflowers, the smell of the damp ground and the trees."

Let go of tension. "Once in the morning and once in the afternoon, I like to close my eyes and take in a nice, deep breath, and as I do, become aware of any tension in my head, scalp and neck," says Dr. Manderino. "Then I let out the air and release any tension that I might have. I take in another breath, become aware of any muscles that might be tight in my head, scalp, neck, shoulders, arms, chest, abdomen and legs, then, as I breathe out, let it go."

Short-circuit negative thinking. "Sometimes I create stress by talking to myself in a way that's critical," says Dr. Manderino. "I'll say, 'That was stupid!' or 'How in the world did you ever get this job?' "

When that happens, "I try to catch myself and correct it immediately. I say, 'Wait a minute—you've had a really busy day, you're really stressed out, no wonder you forgot such and such.' In other words, I take the time to say something in response to my negative thoughts and actually dispute them with a positive statement."

Break free of draining relationships. "As women, all of us can name people who suck the life's blood right out of us," says Dr. Manderino. "They are energy drainers, and it's very important to set limits with them. In some instances, we may have to leave them out of our lives entirely.

"Focus instead on people who are good to you and give you energy," says Dr. Manderino. Spend time with people who are nurturing rather than toxic.

Wait well. Waiting in lines at supermarkets, banks, restaurants

and photocopiers can be very stressful, especially when you're thinking of the 1,001 other things you could be doing.

But don't let it get to you, says Dr. Manderino. "If I'm waiting in a
supermarket line, for instance, instead of letting myself think things
like, 'O-o-o-o-oh, I *hate* waiting in line!,' which is very stressful, I'll do
something else: If there isn't anybody looking, I'll look at one of those
trashy magazines. Or I'll engage in a fantasy."

The Workplace Revolution

Although there are no reptilian dinosaurs roaming the workplace
today, there are tremendous changes there that many workers perceive as equally threatening.

Fueled by global economic expansion and the tremendous economic changes of the 1990s, some American corporations are aban-
doning antiquated management theories left over from the time when
no worker was trusted to work on his own and a "supervisor" was the
guy who flogged the slaves.

The result? "Midlevel management as we know it is going away,"
says organizational psychologist James Campbell Quick, Ph.D., professor of organizational behavior at the University of Texas at Arling-
ton and editor of the *Journal of Occupational Health Psychology*. It's
being replaced by workers who have been organized into teams and
"empowered" to work on their own.

In corporations where this type of organization has been in place,
results have been positive, says Dr. Quick. "Stress levels of both management and workers go down."

Unfortunately, any major workplace changes cause uncertainty
among the workforce, and uncertainty causes stress, says Dr. Quick.
Here are some of the ways a woman can prevent as much stress as
possible from a changing workplace.

Build a nurturing network. One of the key elements in reducing
workplace stress is to build a support system that will nurture you,
says Dr. Quick. And for women, that can mean pulling together a
group of women with common problems and concerns.

In-depth interviews with top male and female executives conducted by Dr. Quick and his colleagues attempted to find out what these highly successful CEOs and CFOs did to reduce stress.

"We looked at everything," says Dr. Quick. "And we found that they didn't all relax, they didn't all play, they didn't all exercise, and they didn't all pray. But what they all *did* do was build social support both in and out of the office."

In particular, female managers got their support from the women who worked for them, says Dr. Quick. The managers formed the nucleus of a group of women that gave the managers the honest feedback and emotional caring they needed. In return, the managers helped the other women develop their work skills. The result was a sense of support for all members of the team—manager and workers alike.

Take control. The less control you have over your work, the more stressed you're likely to feel, says Dr. Quick. But be realistic about what you can and cannot control in a corporate setting. "You can control your own behavior, thinking and response," he says. But you cannot control whether the economy improves, a building starts going up or orders for steel start pouring in.

Sort out your responsibility. Figure out what you are and are not responsible for and don't let people dump unrelated tasks on your plate, says Dr. Quick. Refer them to someone else.

Stay ahead of the steamroller. As the economy continues to evolve over the next decade or so, so will your workplace, says Dr. Quick. And the best way to keep your stress levels low is to position yourself to take advantage of the changes.

"Try to understand what's going on and figure out how you're going to fit into the new structure," says Dr. Quick. "Ask yourself, 'How can I add value to the new organization? Do I need new skills?' "

Then go out and equip yourself to meet the workplace's evolving needs by taking courses, attending workshops or even playing around with new technology related to your field.

Know when to go. When you begin to sense that it's time to move on, do. Otherwise you'll create high stress levels in yourself and those around you.

The Fine Art of Delegation

Superwoman is dead. So stop trying to do it all and let others lend a hand.

Scene I: It's 4:00 P.M. Cynthia Bero, 37, vice-president of an international healthcare consulting firm in Boston, looks at the mountain of projects on her desk. Somehow they all have to be completed within the next few weeks. She knows she should farm them out to her staff, but the mere idea of having to explain everything, of the possible confrontation if the work doesn't meet her standards, exhausts her. Sighing, she reaches for the phone to say she'll be home late again.

Scene II: It's 7:30 A.M. Karen Clark, 36, races into the kitchen. She has two kids to get off to school before her first appointment at the software development company she owns in Knoxville, Tennessee. But as her feet hit the wood floor, her shoes stick to peanut butter from yesterday's lunch. "Why am I the only one who notices this? Doesn't my husband think it's gross?" she fumes. "And why is everything in this house my responsibility?" She quickly mops the floor, her pulse racing while the clock ticks, ticks, ticks . . . .

These women are living at breakneck speed. At home, at work, they go nonstop. Where are their employees, assistants, husbands and kids? Actually, they're right there, ready, able and (mostly) willing to lighten their loads. Yet Bero and Clark, like millions of other women, won't or just can't delegate.

By now we all know that delegating—at home, at work, at the PTA—is critical to reducing stress. "You might have a life, but that life consists of work," says Jo-Ann Abbate, president of About Face Organizers, a productivity and performance consultancy in Stamford, Connecticut. And yes, we know that stress is a killer, that it puts us at greater risk for migraines, insomnia, depression and panic attacks. So why don't we delegate more? We've all heard the stock answer a million times—that girls are socialized to cater to others, boys to be aggressive—but there are other reasons—myths, really—that are just as hard to overcome. Read on.

Five Myths That Keep You Swamped

Myth 1: "It's easier to do it myself." When you're swamped, the thought of teaching someone else how to do something, of making sure they do it right, seems like one more burden. Like Bero, many women dig in and do it themselves instead.

Truth: First, understand that no manager has ever succeeded by doing all the work herself. As Abbate points out, "If you are always the one doing everything, you will always be restricted by what your two hands can achieve. By delegating, you not only increase your productivity, you multiply it."

Next, get past the idea that teaching others takes too much time. "It's a short-term investment for a long-term payoff," says Kay Cronkite Waldo, author of *About Time!: A Women's Guide to Time Management*. "Once your delegatee has learned the job, it's off your shoulders forever."

Myth 2: "It won't get done right if I don't do it." You're convinced that you are the only one who can get this job done properly. Others don't have your expertise, or worse, their standards are considerably lower than yours.

Truth: "That's your ego talking," says Bob Nelson, author of *Empowering Employees through Delegation*. "Are you really the only one smart enough, fast enough, creative enough?" Delegating actually improves the quality of work. When you have several unstressed people working toward a goal, the work will be in much better shape than if one overwhelmed person tries to put out 15 different fires.

"Managers need to remember that their job is delegating. They are there to oversee a project, not do it all," says Bruce Mills, assistant professor of management at the University of Wisconsin School of Business in Madison. Even if your assistant doesn't have your training and foresight, if you don't use his talents, he won't get the practice he needs to bring his work up to snuff. And if you criticize your troops—at work or at home—you'll soon demoralize and lose them. As one husband says, "I'm willing to do my part around the house, but if my efforts are just going to get picked at, then forget it. She can do it all."

Myth 3: "I'll look like a witch." "Despite all the strides we've made in the past few decades, many women are still afraid that by being direct in a request, they risk a confrontation and won't be liked," says Harriet Braiker, Ph.D., author of *The Type E Woman*. This leads some to give muddy instructions ("I feel awful asking you to do this, but if it's not too much trouble, would you mind . . . ?") and others to overcompensate by coming on like Attila the Hun, making their fear of confrontation a self-fulfilling prophecy.

Truth: Those who do the Dance of Nice are so tentative and unclear in their requests that others have no idea what is expected when. The commandos turn people off completely. Why should they do anything for someone who treats them like pond scum? People appreciate receiving precise instructions, and if they are treated reasonably and respectfully, most enjoy the chance to help out or take on a new challenge.

Myth 4: "It's cheating to ask for help." The Superwoman myth lives on. "Women still feel guilty asking for help because we feel we should be able to do everything single-handedly. If we can't, then we're inadequate," says Dr. Braiker. Liz Hartman, 36, director of publicity for a publishing company, admits that despite her demanding schedule, "I feel I must be the one to make play dates and arrange for babysitters. If my husband does it, it means I can't handle the responsibility of both work and child rearing. I've failed."

Truth: Delegating isn't getting other people to do your work, it's figuring out solutions to get projects successfully completed, says Nelson.

Myth 5: "I shouldn't have to tell them, they should know." That's exactly what Clark was thinking, for the umpteenth time, as she swabbed the peanut butter off the floor.

Truth: It would be nice if the people around us were on our exact wavelength, but "that's the fantasy of mental telepathy," says Georgia Witkin, Ph.D., director of the stress program at Mount Sinai School of Medicine in New York City. "People can't possibly know what you want until you tell them. It's that simple."

Direct, Don't Dump

Decided to give delegating a shot? Follow these tips.

Decide what you want to farm out. As a rule, turn over any work that hinders your management of the complete project. The whole point of delegating is to free you from the minutiae so you can oversee the big picture. You should be the one setting the goals; let others execute them.

Don't just dump the grunt work, though: "If you grab all the plum projects, your staff never develops, morale goes down, and it's often not the best use of your time," says Hartman.

Figure out whose help you want. Is there someone especially knowledgeable in this area? Or someone very eager to learn? Clark taught her daughter how to make her bed when she was barely four: "She loved the feeling of accomplishment, and it helped streamline the morning rush." And don't overlook the obvious: hiring someone to help out.

Don't dictate. When you're ready to make the assignment, try to have a conversation about the project with your designated hitter. "When I have a dialogue, I find the other person is better informed and more revved up about the work than if I just barked out an order," says Hartman. If you're anxious about giving direction, Dr. Braiker suggests writing a script and rehearsing it until you're comfortable.

Don't get sidetracked. "If you aren't clear and straightforward in your instructions, you're setting up people for failure," Nelson says. Explain exactly what needs to be accomplished and why; give a due date and a sense of priority if it's a multilayered project. Make sure they know what resources are available to them. "Then have them repeat the assignment back to you so you know they're on track," Nelson says.

If the person you are delegating to is your husband, the process should be very different. You can't give him orders because it puts you in the position of being his boss or mother, not his partner. For true democracy, draw up a list of chores, then hash out who will do what. You may need to renegotiate from time to time, but that's still better than becoming head nudge.

Notify others when you've delegated responsibility. If you ask your teenager to pick up his sister at day care, for example, make sure the teacher is expecting him, or he'll probably return empty-handed.

Don't hover. If you're all over your helpers like glue on flypaper, you haven't freed yourself up at all. Also, your constant interference will undermine their confidence and thus their ability to perform. As long as they reach the desired goal, it doesn't matter what road they take. But don't abandon them, either: They need some guidance and the reassurance that you're there if problems arise. As a safeguard, set up checkpoints to monitor progress: "Let's meet again on Friday to see how you're coming along."

Don't grovel your thanks. Once the project is successfully completed, refrain from simpering, "Oh, thank you, you're a gift from heaven." A simple "You did a great job" will do. If the project fell short, say so in a noncritical way. Adopt a teaching mode while reviewing what went wrong. If you're too harsh, people will hesitate before trying anything new again and you'll be back to your solo act. "Remember: It's a learning process for you and them," cautions Waldo. "It won't go smoothly every time."

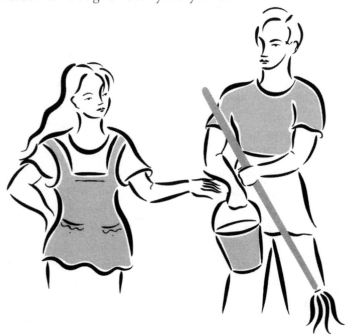

How to Make Up Your Mind

*Stop waffling: Deciding to decide can
actually lower anxiety.*

*m*y sister is the classic decision-phobe. Not long ago, she
called me at 6:45 in the morning to ask my opinion about
a dilemma her tone indicated was of pressing importance—a matter
of national-security proportions. It involved . . . wallpaper.

"I was at the Price and Pack wholesaler's last night," she prattled,
"and I just couldn't decide. The champagne-colored border would
look perfect with my drapes, but the chartreuse pattern would pick
up the trim in my bedspread. So I bought both. Which do you think I
should return?"

I cast my vote, but she remained unconvinced. Next, she called
our other sister, our mom, a friend, her husband, another friend. As it
turned out, she wound up storing both borders in the closet (in case
she changed her mind) and painting the entire room purple! Go
figure.

Despite what you may think, my sister isn't insane—or alone.
Daily decision making is an exercise in frustration for many people.
After all, most of us want to control what we can—and learn to fear
what we can't control. "The unknown really frightens us," explains
Baruch Fischhoff, Ph.D., a psychologist at Carnegie Mellon University
in Pittsburgh. "And the full effect of *any* decision is at the very least
somewhat unknown."

But we can conquer our fear. The trick lies in weighing the
importance—and scariness—of the unknown. "It's natural to experience a certain amount of anxiety when making more complicated life
decisions," says Dr. Fischhoff. "For instance, if we didn't carefully
contemplate whether to relocate for a job or buy that house, we'd be
forfeiting any control we do have over our lives—which isn't normal
or healthy." But neither is fretting unduly over wallpaper patterns.
Balance is the key.

All wafflers do not waffle alike, however. Following are descriptions of five vacillating styles and the steps you can take to change them. Search for your pattern among the five, then choose to change it with conviction.

The Obsessor

The problem: You're a perfectionist who's driven by control, obsessing over decisions large and small. You hem and haw over the finest detail, the faintest wrinkle, and you have a stronger than normal fear of failure. The result: You become so carried away with the process of decision making that you lose sight of the big picture—and your peace of mind.

The solution: "The Obsessor must realize that no matter how much information she has, she cannot possibly *guarantee* the outcome of any decision," says Meredith E. Drench, Ph.D., a health and behavior counselor in East Greenwich, Rhode Island. "So she needs to move on—she has to decide to decide."

As an obsessor, you need to learn to weigh a decision's importance against the amount of time and energy you'll spend contemplating it—and to stop when you strike a balance. Easier said than done? Not really. Simply try this exercise.

Before you make a decision, give yourself a limited amount of time to spend on it. Consider the quandary of choosing between a theme of bunnies or bears for the baby's room. If you allot yourself a week or two in which to decide and two months pass before you even come close to making your choice, you can be sure that you're obsessing—in which case you should forget the bunnies and the bears, and get a grip!

The Waffler

The problem: Like my sister, you seesaw dizzyingly between options. You hound everyone you know for advice, then never take it. You stall, until pressed—at which point you whip yourself into a frenzy and make an impulsive, nonsensical decision to free yourself of your wavering.

The solution: If you think you're a waffler, get into the habit of putting your thoughts on paper, says Diane Halpern, Ph.D., professor of psychology at California State University at San Bernardino and author of the book *Thought and Knowledge: An Introduction to Critical Thinking*. Making a list of pros, cons and consequences associated with each decision will help you to weigh your options more accurately— to focus on one viable solution, instead of innumerable possibilities.

The Passive Ponderer

The problem: You're the queen of passive-aggressive behavior. Paralyzed by the fear of making the "wrong" decision, you forfeit all control—and never make any decisions. You appear ambivalent about your alternatives (even though you care much more than you let on) and you allow them to boil indefinitely—until they erupt in your face.

The solution: You need to shock yourself out of limbo-land, to face your fear of the unknown by conjuring up a worst-case scenario—then choosing with conviction based on the fact that you fully understand the circumstances and that you can survive your decision no matter what the outcome. As a Passive Ponderer, you must ask yourself critical questions such as these whenever you're faced with a decision (an exercise Dr. Drench calls mirroring): So what if you do move in with your boyfriend and it doesn't work out? You can always move out. What are you really afraid of? That you don't really love him enough to seriously consider the next step—the "M" word—and that your doubts will become apparent if you live together? If so, perhaps you should reconsider the relationship itself, not cohabitation.

The Second-Guesser

The problem: No matter how much time and energy you put into a decision, you doubt yourself afterward. (Because it's always your fault.) If the outcome didn't unfold as you had planned, you beat yourself up. (Because it's always your fault.) You dread failure. (Because it's always your fault.)

"Women worry far too much about how their decisions will affect the people around them—their husbands, children, parents, friends and bosses," says Harriette Kaley, Ph.D., a clinical psychologist and psychoanalyst in New York City. "This gives us more reason than men

DECIDING TO DECIDE

*N*o matter what your decision-making style, you can make smart choices. Simply follow these universal rules to making definitive decisions.

Do your homework. If a car salesman tells you he can give you the best interest rate around on a car loan, don't take his word for it. Call several banks to double-check.

Find decisive friends. Consult friends and associates who approach decision making differently. "They can shed a new light on your scenario and help you to get an objective viewpoint," says Baruch Fischhoff, Ph.D., a psychologist at Carnegie Mellon University in Pittsburgh.

Get creative. Think up new solutions to your dilemma. So maybe you can't take the new position because it doesn't pay enough. Perhaps you can do some freelance consulting for the company while you keep your current job. Then, if the right position opens up in the future, you'll already have your foot in the door.

Take calculated risks. If the man you're thinking of marrying has broken off three previous engagements, chances are you won't be his one and only forever. Saying yes might be a risky decision.

Listen to your inner voice. After you've done all your fact-finding, let your psyche take over. "Explore your subconscious for the really important decisions," says Harriette Kaley, Ph.D., a clinical psychologist and psychoanalyst in New York City. "Sleep on your dilemma. Let yourself dream about it. You'd be surprised how a decision can crystallize overnight when you let your intuition take over."

Don't second-guess yourself. Avoid judging your decisions by their outcomes. "A good decision is one in which you made an informed choice with the information you had at the time," says Dr. Fischhoff.

have to doubt ourselves and to feel guilty about our choices."

Our people-pleasing consciences aside, however, women have trouble making decisions for another reason—we generally aren't socialized to be decisive. "We're instructed at a very young age that it's feminine to need help and to solicit advice, answers and affirmation from others," says Dr. Kaley. Women are taught to concern themselves with doing 'the right thing' for other people before doing what's right for them, she says.

Where does this leave us? In dire need of a dose of machismo—that is, confidence. "Men generally take the outcome of their decisions in stride," explains Dr. Kaley. "They instinctively assume that they made the best decision they could at the time and don't blame themselves for decisions gone bad." Women should strive to do the same.

The solution: Stop looking for affirmation from those close to you. Instead, worry about making decisions that meet *your* needs (if you're happy, chances are the people around you will be happy, too). If a choice goes sour, brush it off and move on. And remember, it's *not* your fault.

The Cocky Chooser

The problem: You make hasty decisions, spend little time analyzing your choices and never look back once you make up your mind because consequences don't concern you. In fact, it never occurs to you that you may have made the wrong decision—you chalk up failed outcomes to fate or other external factors.

The solution: The Cocky Chooser "needs to realize that it's good to weigh all the sides of an issue and to think about the various consequences associated with each decision," explains Dr. Drench. "What's more, she needs to take other people's feelings into account, consult others for their opinions and then really listen to what those people have to say."

As a Cocky Chooser, you must also try to learn from your past mistakes. One of the best ways to do this is to keep a decision diary so that you are forced to acknowledge the decisions you've made that may have been hasty or poorly planned. Ask yourself: Did I look at the company thoroughly enough before I took the job? Did I ask my landlubber mate for his opinion before springing for that summer cruise?

"Work hard to build a delay factor—a period of deliberation—into your decision-making process," says Dr. Drench. "This will give you time to run through all the factors surrounding your decision and make sure you haven't overlooked anything."

—*Maureen Boland*

Ten Ways to Take Five

Quick, easy, inexpensive ways to melt tension in 5 to 30 minutes.

*L*et's face it: We all get a little stressed out once in a while. The car breaks down, a check gets bounced, a deadline is missed. Fortunately, these are usually isolated incidents, and when the crisis ends, our brow unfurrows, our breathing slows, our fists unclench and life goes on, relatively free of tension. At least that's the way it's supposed to work.

But sometimes the first crisis is followed by a second . . . and a third. And it's this style of prolonged stress that can run you down, create bags under your eyes and, worst of all, shorten your life span.

Now, here's the good news: You can stop the stress and, in doing so, increase your chances of a long, healthy life.

Surefire Stress Stoppers

Think you might benefit from trying a few tension-taming tactics? Here are ten that the experts recommend.

Lean on a friend. Open up to a loved one about your troubles. Share your hopes, dreams, needs and frustrations. And allow others to do the same with you. Psychologists believe that not only does such intimacy immediately reduce stress, but it also provides loving, nonjudgmental support, which will help give you the confidence you need to deal with your setbacks in a positive manner.

Say a prayer. This can be a very effective way to evoke the stress-relieving relaxation response. Herbert Benson, M.D., associate professor of medicine at Deaconess Hospital in Boston, taught patients the following relaxation method: Find a quiet place and sit comfortably, then choose a soothing word or phrase and repeat it over and over in your mind. "Eighty percent of my patients chose a word or prayer associated with their faith, even though they were offered the choice of other soothing words, such as peace or ocean," says Dr. Benson. And those people who used words related to their religion stayed with the program longer and improved their health more than those who used nonreligious terms.

Soak away your stress. Experts say that warm baths help alleviate tension not only by relaxing your muscles, but also by slightly heating your brain, which can be calming. The temperature of the bathwater should be comfortably warm to the touch—between 100° and 102°F. (If the water's too hot it can shock your system and cause your muscles to constrict.) And if you have a heart condition be sure to limit your soaking time to 15 minutes or less; longer tubbing could cause your blood pressure to drop, and you could faint.

Get a pet. A dog, cat or even a fish can be a faithful friend who'll listen to your troubles—and maybe even save your life. Research has shown that heart attack victims who have pets live longer. What's more, watching a tankful of tropical fish may lower blood pressure—at least temporarily. Also, pets may relieve stress by bringing out our more playful side and making us smile.

Laugh it off. If you're caught in a situation that you can't escape from or change, humor may be the healthiest form of release from your temporary stress. During the laugh itself, your heart rate and blood pressure rise slightly, after which there's an immediate release—your muscles relax and your blood pressure sinks below pre-laugh levels. A good giggle may also prompt the brain to emit endorphins, the same stress-reducing biochemicals that are triggered by exercise. And a hearty chuckle can even help fight illness by temporarily boosting your body's level of immunoglobulin A, a virus-fighting antibody.

Listen to the blues. Or jazz. Or classical. Whatever the reason, music helps relieve stress. Studies show that music played for patients before, during and after surgery seems to decrease the feelings of surgery-associated stress by reducing the amount of stress hormones secreted in the brain. "Even after the music is turned off, the mind continues to reduce the patients' anxiety and pain," says Fred Schwartz, M.D., an anesthesiologist at Piedmont Hospital in Atlanta. "This enables the anesthesiologist to administer fewer sedatives before, during and after the surgery." So when stress strikes, turn on the tunes that you find most comforting.

Picture a tranquil scene. Dew shimmers on rose petals at sunrise. Waves roll lazily onto a steamy tropical beach. Although scientists don't yet know why, envisioning pleasant scenes such as these can help you become the picture of tranquillity. One study revealed that hospital patients whose rooms overlooked trees recovered faster than those who viewed a brick wall. If you don't find yourself in or near any real-life tranquil settings, try gazing at a photograph of one. Then focus on enjoying the serenity of the setting just as you would if you were there.

Take a hike. When you're stressed, your body releases adrenalin to prepare your body to fight or flee. To get rid of this excess adrenalin, you need to get moving—to, in essence, flee.

That's where walking comes in. Walking instantly helps dissipate this chemical. But you don't have to wait for stress to strike to hit the high road: You can also take a stroll to avoid a stressful situation or to clear your mind before facing an inevitable one. Or take a walking break at work to escape a boring routine and reinvigorate yourself. In addition to alleviating existing stress, regular walking helps to condition your body so that future stressful events will take less of a toll.

Breathe easy. "Deep breathing is one of the simplest yet most effective stress-management techniques there is," says Dean Ornish, M.D., president and director of the Preventive Medicine Research Institute in Sausalito, California. Breathing deeply works by infusing the blood with extra oxygen and causing the body to release endorphins, your body's natural tranquilizing hormones.

To take a relaxing breath, slowly inhale through your nose, expanding your abdomen before allowing air to fill your chest. Then

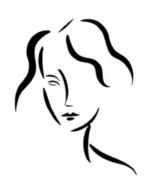

slowly exhale. Practice this for a few minutes each day or whenever stress strikes.

Focus your attention. Allow your mind to become fixed on a pleasant sight, sound or smell. It can be the sight of clouds floating by, the sound of a bird singing outside or the aroma of bread baking. Focus on the image, sound or smell, allowing your mind to be free of all other thoughts for a few moments. Be sure to take time for a few mental rest stops throughout the day.

Positive Strokes

Massage unkinks knotted muscles and actually helps reduce the body's level of stress hormones. (And it feels so good.)

A massage may seem like a luxury that requires more time and money than you have. But when you consider its benefits, which range from dekinked muscles to improved self-esteem, massage begins to seem worth the money. Think of massage as a tiny spa vacation, and you'll get the idea.

The Power of Touch

What is it exactly that makes a professional massage so rewarding? To most of us, it simply feels good to be touched. But massage isn't just touch; it's touch applied with pressure, and that's key. The pressure, say massage researchers, helps reduce the body's level of stress hormones. "We don't think touch works the same way without pressure, probably because pressure stimulates certain sensory receptors that light touch doesn't," says Tiffany Field, Ph.D., director of the University of Miami School of Medicine's Touch Research Institute.

In one recent study, massage treatments dramatically relieved back pain in 86 percent of patients. "The usual methods for treating pain, heat and ultrasound, don't get down deep enough to get to the source of the pain," says Michael I. Weintraub, M.D., clinical professor of neurology at New York Medical College in Valhalla, who conducted the study. "The only way to do that is manually."

Studies have also shown that massage increases the blood flow, which helps hasten the removal of metabolic waste products such as lactic acid, one of the main culprits behind sore muscles. Massage can also reduce muscle tightness—making you feel as if you'd had a good stretch, but better—and has been shown to stimulate the release of endorphins, brain chemicals that are the body's natural painkillers.

The pleasure of a massage, though, may be as much psychological as physical. "Massage communicates a sense of acceptance," says Martha Brown Menard, a massage therapist and researcher at the University of Virginia in Charlottesville, who is investigating the role of massage in recovering from surgery. "Most people feel self-conscious about their bodies, but when someone touches them, it's like saying, 'You're okay, your body's okay,' no matter what shape it's in." As one woman puts it, "I feel beautiful every time I get a massage."

So why not just cajole your husband into giving you a back rub—or at least bribe the kids to rub your feet? Nice as these things can be (though they too usually have a price), a professional offers a level of expertise that little-kid hands and even loving-husband hands can't. "Massage therapists are trained to understand things like pinched nerves and muscle tears, problems that an untrained person can exacerbate," says Myk Hungerford, Ph.D., director of the American Institute of Massage Therapy in Costa Mesa, California. "They are also trained to understand referred pain—meaning that the muscle that hurts isn't necessarily the one that needs to be worked on." (The term *massage therapist*, by the way, is a sign of the times. As the industry tries to shed the sexual connotations associated with massage, the words *masseuse* and *masseur* have become passé.)

Which Rub Is for You?

There are practically as many kinds of massage as there are massage therapists. The most prevalent is Swedish massage, which involves long strokes and the kneading of muscles. But some therapists also throw in a little shiatsu, or acupressure techniques based on

FIVE TIP-OFFS THAT YOU KNEAD A MASSAGE

*B*elow are five sure-fire signs that you could use a massage, according to Isadora Guggenheim, a licensed massage therapist in New York.

You're lethargic. You're not lazy, you're stressed out. Massage releases the fatigue from your muscles and puts the bounce back in your step.

Your shoulders are up near your ears. If tension has rearranged your shoulders or made your hips so crooked your skirts don't hang straight, you need to be kneaded.

You have lower back pain. This is not nerve pain (which is searing and unrelenting) but a deep, dull ache. A pro can coax those muscles out of spasm.

You're an exerciser. Whether you're a marathoner or a weekend athlete, a massage before or after exercise will increase your flexibility and keep you limber.

You need to be touched. Cats, dogs and kids are smart—they know they need their daily quota of touch. So do you. If there's no one in your life to hold you right now, try a therapeutic laying on of hands.

the Chinese idea of energy channels, or meridians, that run throughout the body. To open these channels, the therapist presses on certain body points, using his or her fingers and sometimes elbows or even feet. "It's similar to acupuncture, but it has a softer needle," says Drew Francis, owner of Golden Cabinet Herbs, an acupuncture and acupressure center in West Los Angeles.

Another technique, trigger-point therapy, is similar to acupressure in that it also involves pressing hypersensitive points that relate to other parts of the body. "There may, for instance, be a spot on the shoulder that relieves the pain in the lower arm," explains Elliot Greene, former president of the American Massage Therapy Association and a therapist in Silver Spring, Maryland.

Sports massage is another up-and-coming technique. Used by professional athletes both before competition (to prep muscles) and after (to soothe them), it's now offered by many spas and salons to ease workout-related aches and pains.

Aromatherapy massages, offered by many salons, usually incorporate Swedish massage techniques with the added bonus of scented oils intended to either relax or invigorate you. (Most massage therapists use lightweight oils that generate warmth and reduce friction. They usually don't leave you greasy, but if a scalp massage is included, you'll want to shampoo afterward.)

Finding a Therapist

No one technique is better than another. All have benefits, and those benefits ultimately hinge on the skill of the person doing the massaging. Massage therapists at a local Y, health club, salon or day spa may have been screened by the organization. But it's still important to ask for credentials (some states license therapists) or to inquire whether the therapist belongs to a professional association or has received at least 500 hours of training at an accredited school. Word of mouth is another good way to find a massage pro, especially a freelance therapist who will come to your home. Or you can call the American Massage Therapy Association at (708) 864-0123 for a recommendation.

But a recommendation is no guarantee that you'll click with a therapist. "Since there are so many different styles, you may have to try a couple of different people before you find the right one," says Greene.

Massage Etiquette: What's Proper, What's Not

When you make an appointment for a massage at a salon or health club, you should be asked whether you prefer a man or a woman (some places automatically assign same-sex therapists to clients). For most massages—acupressure and shiatsu are sometimes exceptions—you'll be stark naked, so if you have reservations about nudity, a woman is probably the better choice. With most therapists, however, you won't feel naked: Expect them to leave the room while you disrobe and to give you a towel or sheet to place over your body. During the massage only the area being worked on will be exposed.

Before the massage starts, the therapist should ask you about your health (if you haven't already filled out a questionnaire in the waiting room) and any aches and pains you might have. Now's the time to mention your stiff neck or sore feet. Now's also the time, if you're not a fan of New Age or classical music, to mention that you'd prefer silence. (You may not have a choice: Many salons pipe mood music into their massage rooms, and you just have to live with it.)

Some massage pros, like some manicurists, are chatty. If you don't want to talk, say so or just keep quiet—most therapists will take the cue from you.

No two massage therapists perform massage in exactly the same way. Some will begin with the front of your body, some with the back. But whatever they do, it shouldn't hurt. Sometimes it takes pressure to work the kinks out of knotty muscles, but the pressure should be bearable. "The therapist might work the muscle right to the edge of discomfort, but not to the point where the muscle begins to tense and fight back," says Deborah Wood, director of Medical Massage Therapy Associates in Colorado Springs, Colorado. After a deep-muscle massage, though, there may be some next-day soreness.

What You'll Pay

Costs vary from city to city. Expect to pay between $35 and $60 for a one-hour massage, plus a 15 percent tip when appropriate. (Extras cost more: Noelle The Day Spa in Stamford, Connecticut, which charges about $60 for a basic massage, also offers a four-handed massage—with two massage therapists—for about $110.)

As with any kind of treatment—say, a facial or a haircut—the benefits of a massage are generally short-term. You'll probably sleep well the night after a massage and feel more relaxed and limber for the next few days. "But if you have massages on a regular basis, the stress-reduction benefits can be long-term," says Greene.

If you're unsure about making the leap to a full body massage, consider a few mini-massage options. Facials, for instance, generally include a head, neck and shoulder rub. Or you can literally dip your toe into massage by having a pedicure, which usually involves a lower leg and foot rub, or possibly a foot reflexology massage, which is a kind of acupressure for the feet.

A Spa of One's Own

No time or money for a spa visit? Re-create the spa experience in the privacy of your own home.

*Y*ou're in the lap of luxury: hands massaging your scalp, hot baths relaxing your tense muscles, scented towels wrapping your warm body. At the end of a rejuvenating day at a spa, your skin glows, your hair shines, your mind's at peace. You're ready for anything—except, perhaps, the bill. It's $300. So much for peace of mind.

But taking time to pamper yourself is a necessity—not a luxury—if you want to look and feel your best. "A spa treatment leaves you not only more beautiful, but also more relaxed and better able to deal with the stresses of daily life," says herbalist Brigitte Mars of Boulder, Colorado.

Alison Howland, a global educator for the body-care products manufacturer Aveda, agrees. "Even though I work in a spa, scheduling time for treatments for myself is almost impossible," she says.

The solution? Both Howland and Mars set aside one night a week for a spa evening at home. "At-home spa days are an opportunity for clearing the body and mind," says Mars, who regularly turns her home into a spa retreat for herself and her husband.

With the high-quality natural bath and beauty products available today, the hot mineral springs bath, aromatherapy treatments and herbal facials offered by the finest health spas can be easily—and affordably—re-created at home. For example, in less than three minutes (and for less than five dollars), you can give yourself a refreshing aromatherapy facial and feel calmer all over. Imagine inhaling lavender or geranium and exhaling the day's worries.

Creating a spa at home also allows you to customize treatments so you can tailor them to your schedule. Once a week or once a month, set aside some time to indulge yourself with a full body treatment, such as a deep-condition hair treatment, followed by a facial sauna, a mask, and a soak in your favorite aromatherapy bath. When time is tight between at-home spa sessions, use the quick treatments every day to boost your mood and revitalize your body.

"The first step is to claim your sacred space," Mars advises. Turn off the phone, hang a Do Not Disturb sign on the door; do whatever it takes to block off an hour or two of uninterrupted time for yourself. You might consider getting together with your partner or a friend to share this nurturing experience. Whatever you decide, prepare for your spa treatment by making sure you have all the necessary ingredients. Then, just relax and enjoy.

Hair and Scalp Therapy

HERBAL FINISHING RINSE

Time Required: Two minutes
What You'll Need: Herbal hair rinse (or herbs and distilled water if you're making your own)

Follow shampoo and conditioner with an herbal rinse to remove any shampoo residue and bring out the natural highlights in your hair. Look for rinses containing herbs such as rosemary, horsetail, sage, lavender, nettles and chamomile. Mars recommends a combination of equal parts of rosemary and nettles for dark hair or chamomile and lemongrass for light hair. To make your own, bring one quart of water and four tablespoons of dried herbs to a boil in a covered pot. Turn off the heat and allow the herbs to steep until cool. Strain out the herbs, and use a half-cup of the infused water as a final rinse. This mixture will stay fresh in the refrigerator for up to one week.

STIMULATING SCALP MASSAGE

Time Required: Three minutes
What You'll Need: Essential oils (rosemary and sage), witch hazel

This easy scalp massage feels great and provides a dose of quick energy. According to aromatherapist Ann Berwick, author of *Holistic Aromatherapy*, some people believe that stimulating oils such as rosemary and sage may even promote hair growth. Berwick recommends using a solution of four drops of rosemary and four drops of sage essential oils with one teaspoon of witch hazel. This invigorating blend can be massaged into the scalp daily, either in the morning or before going to bed. A few drops can also be sprinkled onto your hairbrush immediately prior to brushing to condition your hair and make it shine.

DEEP-CONDITIONING HAIR TREATMENT

Time Required: 30 minutes
What You'll Need: Jojoba oil, rosemary and sage essential oils, a shower cap

Once a week, treat your hair and scalp to a deep-conditioning treatment to combat the damage caused by overcleansing, heat and chemical treatments. In a small container combine one teaspoon of jojoba oil with four drops of rosemary and four drops of sage essential oils. Massage this mixture into your scalp with your fingertips. If your scalp tends to be oily, apply this only to the ends of your hair. When applied, put on a shower cap and let the oils remain in your hair for 30 minutes. (This is an ideal time to indulge in a spa bath treatment.) Follow this treatment with a shampoo—lather twice to remove the oil—and conditioner if needed.

Facials That Refresh

"Avoid becoming locked into a skin-care routine," says Howland. Why? Because your skin is always changing. The outer layer, or epidermis, is replaced approximately every 28 days. As a result, minor variations in the way that you care for your skin can produce dramatically different results. For example, exfoliating your skin regularly eliminates dead skin cells and gives your complexion a fresher, smoother appearance. In addition, your skin is constantly changing as your body changes with your diet, exercise, age and even the seasons. Watch for these changes in your skin, and choose products and treatments accordingly.

CLEANSING

Time Required: Two minutes
What You'll Need: Cleanser suited to your skin type, washcloth

Cleansing removes the day's accumulations of dirt and makeup, plus the waste products excreted by the skin. It's important to choose a cleanser formulated for your particular skin type. Cleansing creams and milks are suitable for dry to normal and sensitive skin. Oil-free gels and foaming cleansers are more appropriate for oily to normal or blemished skin. Soap has a tendency to cause dryness, but if you feel you must use it on your face, look for one that contains soothing ingredients such as honey, chamomile, oatmeal, calendula or goat's milk.

To cleanse your skin, moisten your face with warm water. Spread a small amount of cleanser over your entire face, making little circular motions with the pads of your fingers. Gently remove the cleanser with a warm washcloth, and rinse thoroughly with warm water. Finish with a splash of cool water.

TONING

Time Required: One minute
What You'll Need: Astringent or toner (witch hazel, essential oils and distilled water if you're making your own), cotton balls

Toners are gentler than astringents and are suitable for all skin types. Soothing ingredients such as rose water, aloe, kelp, chamomile, lavender, calendula, cucumber and comfrey are combined to make natural toners.

To make your own simple toner, Berwick suggests mixing one-half teaspoon of witch hazel with the essential oils appropriate for your skin type (see the instructions under "Aromatherapy Facial Steam" below) in a four-ounce bottle. Shake vigorously to dissolve the essential oils in the witch hazel, and fill the bottle with distilled water. This toner will need to be shaken before each use. Apply one-half teaspoon onto a cotton ball, and gently wipe it over your skin. Toners can also be placed into a spray bottle and spritzed onto your skin several times during the day as a quick refresher and skin hydrator.

MOISTURIZING

Time Required: 30 seconds
What You'll Need: Moisturizer of your choice (or jojoba and other essential oils if you're making your own)

Moisturizing your skin immediately after applying toner, while the skin is still damp, will help hold water in the skin. Water, not oil, is what keeps the skin plump and moist. Choose a moisturizer appropriate for your skin type. Dry skin responds well to moisturizers containing heavy plant oils such as cocoa and karite butters, while oily skin benefits more from lighter moisturizers such as aloe vera.

To make a simple facial moisturizer, Berwick suggests adding the essential oils appropriate for your skin type to jojoba oil. Add ten drops of essential oil to one ounce of jojoba oil. Mist your face first with toner, and then massage three or four drops of the oil onto damp skin.

SKIN-REFINING EXFOLIATION

Time Required: Three minutes
What You'll Need: Facial scrub (oats, cornmeal or almonds, and honey if you're making your own), washcloth

Facial exfoliants remove the accumulation of dead cells that cause skin to look flaky or dull; they are one of the quickest treatments for improving the appearance of your skin. The simplest exfoliants are made from finely ground grains and nuts such as oatmeal, cornmeal, almonds, apricot kernels and walnuts.

To make your own facial scrub, Mars suggests combining two parts of finely ground rolled oats with one part of finely ground cornmeal. People with dry or sensitive skin should replace the cornmeal with finely ground almond meal. Mix two teaspoons of the scrub with one teaspoon of honey, and gently massage it onto damp skin. When finished, rinse your face with warm water. A gentle facial scrub can be used daily for oily or normal skin, and two or three times a week for dry skin.

DEEP-CLEANSING FACIAL SAUNA

Time Required: 25 minutes
What You'll Need: Distilled or spring water, herbs, large pot with lid, towel

Spa facials invariably include a facial sauna to open the pores, deep-cleanse the skin and bring a healthy glow to the complexion. This treatment can easily be replicated at home with a steaming pot of fragrant herbs. Herbal blends made especially for facial steams are available at natural food stores, or you can create your own. Mars suggests using equal parts of comfrey, calendula and rose for dry skin;

lemongrass, orange peel and rosemary for oily skin; and calendula, peppermint and chamomile for normal skin.

To prepare a facial sauna, bring two quarts of water and four to six tablespoons of herbs to a boil in a large covered pot. Turn off the heat and allow the herbs to steep for ten minutes. Place the pot on a table, remove the lid and make a towel tent over both your head and the steaming pot. Stay under the tent for ten minutes to allow your pores to open and perspiration to deep-cleanse your skin. Follow this by splashing your face with warm, and then cool, water.

AROMATHERAPY FACIAL STEAM
Time Required: 15 minutes
What You'll Need: Distilled or spring water, heat-proof bowl, essential oils, towel

Essential oils can be used to create a simple and fragrant aromatherapy facial steam. Pour 1½ quarts of boiling water into a large, heat-proof bowl. Add the essential oils according to your skin type, and make a tent over your head and the bowl with a large towel. Breathe deeply, and remain under the towel for ten minutes. Berwick suggests the following combinations of essential oils for facial steams.

Normal skin: Two drops lavender or geranium
Sensitive skin: Two drops chamomile or lavender
Oily skin: Two drops juniper or tea tree (especially helpful for blemishes)
Dry skin: Two drops sandalwood or patchouli
Mature skin: Two drops lavender or frankincense

AROMATHERAPY HOT TOWEL FACIAL
Time Required: Three minutes
What You'll Need: Essential oils, washcloth

For a quick cleansing treatment when you don't have time for a full-fledged facial steam, Howland suggests an aromatherapy hot towel treatment. Begin by washing your skin as usual. Add two drops of lavender or geranium essential oil to a basin of hot water. Soak a small hand towel or washcloth in the scented hot water, wring out the cloth and apply it to your face for a minute or two.

MOISTURIZING MASK

Time Required: 25 minutes
What You'll Need: Moisturizing mask treatment (or avocado and yogurt if you're making your own), washcloth

Dry, normal and mature skin types benefit from weekly moisturizing mask treatments. For a rich mask that will leave your skin soft and dewy, combine one-quarter of a very ripe avocado and one teaspoon of yogurt. Mix them well and apply to clean skin. Remove it after 20 minutes with a warm, wet washcloth.

The Ultimate Bath

Soaking in a special bath is the ultimate at-home spa experience. Wonderfully versatile, baths can soothe, detoxify or energize, depending on the ingredients and water temperature you select. Begin by creating a special atmosphere: A thick, soft towel and cozy robe are essentials. Soothing music and fragrant candles add to the ambiance; a cup of herbal tea can enhance the desired effects of the bath. *Note:* Use caution when using oils in the bath because they make the tub slippery. Use a rubber tub mat for safety.

PREBATH CIRCULATION-STIMULATING BODY BRUSHING

Time Required: Five minutes
What You'll Need: A natural bristle body brush or a loofah

While running your bath, take a few minutes to brush your skin with a natural bristle body brush or a dry loofah. This gentle massage stimulates circulation and removes dead cells from the surface of your skin. Brush with gentle strokes, beginning with the bottoms of your feet, moving up your legs, hips and abdomen, then up your arms from fingertips to shoulders, across your torso and back, and finishing with your neck. Follow this by sinking into the bath of your choice.

RELAXING BATH

Time Required: 20 to 45 minutes
What You'll Need: Your choice of relaxing bath herbs, washcloth, string,
herbal tea, essential oils, vegetable oil or whole milk, bath or Epsom salts

For a simple herbal bath, tie a handful of herbs into a washcloth and secure them with a piece of string. Place this ball of herbs into the tub while the hot water is running. To make your own calming bath blend, combine equal parts of chamomile, lavender and linden flowers. Sipping a cup of fragrant chamomile or linden flower tea while soaking will enhance the relaxing effect of the bath.

Aromatherapy essential oils can also be used to promote deep relaxation. "An aromatherapy bath is one of the best ways to 'de-stress,' " says Howland. The benefits of essential oils go far beyond their pleasing aromas. Essential oils retain the healing properties of the herbs and flowers from which they are distilled. During a warm bath, the vapors are inhaled; the oils are absorbed through the skin and are circulated throughout the body by the bloodstream. Relief from anxiety and stress, headaches, muscle tension and premenstrual syndrome are just a few of the benefits attributed to aromatherapy.

Berwick suggests the following simple aromatherapy bath for relaxation: Dilute four drops of lavender, two drops of clary sage and two drops of marjoram in one teaspoon of vegetable oil such as almond oil or one teaspoon of whole milk. (Most essential oils must be diluted in another oil to prevent possible skin irritation.) Fill the tub with hot water (use warm water if you have circulatory problems), and add the diluted essential oils just before getting in.

To increase the relaxing effect of your bath, add mineral bath salts (available at natural food stores) or one cup of Epsom salts to the tub. Most mineral bath treatments include Epsom salts, which contains magnesium sulfate. Magnesium promotes deep relaxation of the muscles and nervous system. To complete your calming bath experience, "let the water run out of the tub when you're finished soaking, and visualize your stress vanishing down the drain as well," suggests Mars.

DETOXIFYING BATH

Time Required: 30 to 45 minutes
What You'll Need: Your choice of essential oils, bath herbs, vegetable oil or whole milk

Many spa treatments are designed to help eliminate toxins from the body. Baths, in particular, aid in detoxification by promoting sweating, and various herbs and essential oils increase circulation and stimulate the functions of the eliminative organs. Look for detoxifying bath products containing herbs and essential oils such as juniper, grapefruit, fennel, dandelion and burdock.

To create your own aromatherapy detoxifying bath, Berwick suggests adding four drops of juniper, two drops of grapefruit and two drops of rosemary to one teaspoon of vegetable oil or whole milk; add this mixture to a tub of hot water. A hot bath is most effective for promoting sweating, but avoid very hot water if you have circulatory problems. Soak in the bath for 20 to 30 minutes.

Credits

"Understanding Urinary Incontinence" was adapted from "Stress Incontinence" by Mary Murray, originally published in *Glamour*. Copyright © 1995 by Mary Murray. Reprinted by permission.

"Thyroid Disease: A Woman's Guide" was adapted from "Recognizing Thyroid Trouble" by Nancy Monson, which originally appeared in *Glamour*. Copyright © 1995 by Nancy Monson. Reprinted by permission.

"Sleep Better, Feel Better" was adapted from "Why You Just Can't Get to Sleep" by Dorothy Foltz-Gray, originally published in *RED-BOOK*. Copyright © 1995 by Dorothy Foltz-Gray. Reprinted by permission.

PART THREE

"Foods That Help Turn Back the Clock" was adapted from "The Healthiest Foods: Are You Eating Enough?" by Peggy Noonan, originally published in *Longevity*. Reproduced by permission of Longevity, copyright © 1995, Longevity International, Ltd.

"The World's Healthiest Diet?" was adapted from "The World's Healthiest Diet" by Bibi Wein, which originally appeared in *SELF*. Copyright © 1995 by Bibi Wein. Reprinted by permission.

"Eat to Energize!" was adapted from *Food and Mood: The Complete Guide to Eating Well and Feeling Your Best* by Elizabeth Somer, M.A., R.D. Copyright © 1995 by Elizabeth Somer. Reprinted by permission of Henry Holt and Co.

PART FOUR

"Two Dozen Ways to De-fat Your Diet" was adapted from "Cook Rich, Eat Light" by Janis Jibrin, R.N., originally published in *Longevity*. Reproduced by permission of Longevity, copyright © 1995, Longevity International, Ltd.

PART FIVE

"A Beginner's Guide to Getting Fit" was adapted from *The Lazy Person's Guide to Fitness* by Charles Swencionis, Ph.D. and E. Davis Ryan, P.T. Copyright © 1994 by Charles Swencionis and E. Davis Ryan. Reprinted by permission of Barricade Books, Inc.

"Yoga: The Gentlest Way to Shape Up" was adapted from "The New Yoga" by Linda Dyett. Courtesy *SELF*. Copyright © 1995 by the Conde Nast Publications, Inc.

PART SIX

"Young Skin for Life" was adapted from "Your Skin" by Laurie Drake, originally published in *SELF*. Copyright © 1994 by Laurie Drake. Reprinted by permission.

"The Sensitive Type" was adapted from "Sensitivity Training for Your Skin." Courtesy *Mademoiselle*. Copyright © 1995 by the Conde Nast Publications, Inc.

"More Than Just Mud" was adapted from "The Wild New Masks" by Kate Staples, which originally appeared in *SELF*. Copyright © 1995 by Kate Staples. Reprinted by permission.

PART SEVEN

"A Better Way to Argue" was adapted from "The Dirty Fighter" by Susan Browder, which originally appeared in *New Woman*. Copyright © 1995 by Susan Browder. Reprinted by permission.

PART EIGHT

"The Fine Art of Delegation" was adapted from "Are You Doing Too Much of the Dirty Work?" by Beth Levine, originally published in *REDBOOK*. Copyright © 1995 by Beth Levine. Reprinted by permission.

"Positive Strokes" was adapted from "Please Touch! The Healing Power of Massage" by Daryn Eller, originally published in *REDBOOK*. Copyright © 1995 by Daryn Eller. Reprinted by permission.

"A Spa of One's Own" was adapted from "The Spa at Home" by Laurel Vukovic. Reprinted with permission from *Natural Health*, March/April 1995. For more information, call 1-800-937-4766.

Index

Note: Underscored page references indicate boxed text. **Boldface** references indicate illustrations and tables.

B